Clinical Governance

Clinical Governance

Making It Happen

Myriam Lugon

Medical Director
Forest Healthcare Trust, Whipps Cross Hospital
London, UK

Jonathan Secker-Walker

Senior Lecturer and Honorary Consultant
University of Wales College of Medicine
Cardiff, UK

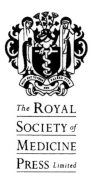

The ROYAL
SOCIETY *of*
MEDICINE
PRESS *Limited*

© 1999 Royal Society of Medicine Press Ltd
Reprinted 1999 (twice)
Reprinted 2000
1 Wimpole Street, London W1M 8AE, UK
207 Westminster Road, Lake Forest, IL, 60045, USA

British Library Cataloguing in Publication Data
A catalogue record for this book is available from the British Library

ISBN 1 85315 383 4

Phototypeset by Phoenix Photosetting, Chatham, Kent
Printed in Great Britain by Bell and Bain Ltd, Glasgow

▶ Contents

▶ List of Contributors

Conor Burke Clinical Risk and Audit Manager, Whipps Cross Hospital, London

Jane Cartwright Clinical Risk Manager, St Mary's Hospital, London

Anne-Louise Ferguson Managing Solicitor, Head of Welsh Health Legal Services, Cardiff

Ewan Ferlie Professor of Public Services Management, Imperial College Management School, Imperial College of Science, Technology and Medicine, London

Julie Glanville Information Service Manager, NHS Centre for Reviews and Dissemination, York

Dorothy Gregson Joint Acting Director of Public Health, Kensington, Chelsea and Westminster Health Authority, London

David Hands Independent Health Services Development Consultant, Kidderminster

Rosemary Hittinger Senior Clinical Audit Coordinator, St Mary's Hospital, London

Susan Hobbs Chief Nurse, University Hospital of Wales, Cardiff

David Ingram Professor of Health Informatics, University College, London

Neil Jackson Dean of Postgraduate General Practice Education, North Thames East, Thames Postgraduate Medical and Dental Education, London

Sue Johnson Independent Consultant, Sue Johnson Associates, Alton

Dipak Kalra Clinical Senior Lecturer in Health Informatics, University College, London

Myriam Lugon Medical Director, Forest Healthcare Trust, Whipps Cross Hospital, London

David Patterson Consultant Physician and Cardiologist, Whittington Hospital, London

Kate Phipps Assistant Director of Nursing, NHS Executive, London Regional Office, London

Marianne Rigge Director, College of Health, London

Jonathan Secker-Walker Senior Lecturer and Honorary Consultant, University of Wales College of Medicine, Cardiff

Jenny Simpson Chief Executive, British Association of Medical Managers, Stockport

Tony Weight Deputy Director of Education and Training, NHS Executive, London Regional Office, London

▶ Preface

Most staff in healthcare have heard about clinical governance but probably wonder what it means for them and their organisation. The term may be new but it covers an approach to quality that we should have all adopted. The book is an attempt to demystify the concept. It addresses the components of governance from the patient's expectations to frameworks for risk and claims management, the role of clinical improvement groups in taking the governance agenda forward and informatics for the millennium. Whilst the organisational responsibility and approach is described, it is recognised that the successful delivery of this agenda depends on the commitment of the workforce and an approach that develops clinical teams. Practical examples are given which may help the reader when thinking through the issues they face in their own organisation. Although this book is not aimed directly at primary care provision, it is likely that many of the suggestions would be applicable to this area. It should be useful for managers, clinical directors, many clinicians and specialist registrars who need to understand what clinical governance means for examination purposes.

Myriam Lugon
Jonathan Secker-Walker
1999

▶1

Introduction

Myriam Lugon and Jonathan Secker-Walker

The editor of the BMJ writing in the aftermath of the Bristol cardiac surgery case[1] used a quotation from WB Yeats, 'All changed, changed utterly:' as his title. Clinical governance will, for the first time, place the quality of care as well as financial probity as the direct responsibility of the Chief Executive, and therefore the Board, of NHS Trusts. It is probably no coincidence that the concept of clinical governance was written into the Government's White Paper *The new NHS. Modern. Dependable*[2] whilst the General Medical Council hearings were underway. The Bristol case was but another in a series of medical disasters relating to cervical screening, breast screening, psychiatric care, histopathological diagnosis and more recently gynae-cology, that have received considerable media coverage and left scores of patients either damaged or with uncertainty. There can be little doubt that if clinicians grasp the opportunity, clinical governance should do much to restore the trust that society and patients have historically had in medicine. Failure to do so will lead to a web of regulations, national databases and constraints on doctors being imposed from outside the profession, similar to the situation suffered by clinicians across the Atlantic.

This book aims to cover some of the aspects of the organisation and function of healthcare that will be directly affected by the introduction of clinical governance. What regular information will the Chief Executive require to be satisfied that the quality of clinical care is adequate? Who will be responsible for collecting the information? How accurate will it be? What systems and processes need to be in place to ensure the quality of care delivery? It is aimed to offer practical tips whenever possible. The book does not, however, cover the implementation of clinical governance in primary care, which may require a different approach, though this will need to be systematic. It is probable that the principles and practical steps described in the various chapters could often be translated to be applicable in primary care settings.

So what is clinical governance? It can be defined as the action, the system or the manner of governing clinical affairs. This requires two main components; an explicit means of setting clinical policy and an equally explicit means of monitoring compliance with such policy.

Clinical policy

Clinical policy is most often agreed at directorate level, and especially where care pathways are used. Such policy is often arrived at by agreeing to adopt – or adapt – a national guideline. However, it would appear likely that the influence of the National

Institute for Clinical Excellence (NICE) and the need to implement recommendations from incident review and risk management committees will require hospitals to have some form of Clinical Policy Committee. This committee would then recommend that certain clinical policies are implemented across the Trust. The issue of clinical freedom, which is to a large extent illusory in a cash limited health service, is beyond the scope of this introduction. However, it would seem from recent medico-legal judgements[3] that clinicians are free to deviate from agreed policies or protocols but need to record their reasons in the medical notes and be prepared to provide a logical argument as to why they have done so.

Most hospitals have several monitoring systems in place already. These, under the old cogwheel organisational structure, had clearly defined reporting routes. Such systems would include committees dealing with infection control, medical records, blood transfusion, radiological protection, drug and therapeutics. With the advent of changed organisational structures (clinical directorates), exactly where these monitoring committees reported and who was responsible for effecting their recommendations has often been unclear. Clinical audit departments are likely to change from a role, at best, tolerated by doctors, to one of monitoring whether or not the recommendations from the National Institute for Clinical Excellence, trust risk management, the committees mentioned above are, in fact, translated into practice. The regular provision to clinical directors of analysis of their trusts' minimum datasets derived from coding at death or discharge will identify outlying performance by consultant and disease or operation code. Since the coded information taken from medical records is the data by which Trusts will be measured for performance, it is clearly in everyone's interest that the standard and clarity of the medical notes facilitates reliable disease and operation coding by the coding staff – which whom regular dialogue will be essential.

Full participation

A first class service. Quality in the new NHS the consultation paper following the Government's White Paper[4] envisages full participation by all hospital doctors in audit programmes, including specialty and subspecialty national external audit programmes endorsed by the Commission for Health Improvement. Whilst some specialties, for instance cardiac surgery, have good national performance data, there are other areas where concise data are not easily available. Comparisons between patient length of stay and outcomes may not be very meaningful where multiple pathology exists in medical or geriatric care or in tertiary referral centres for complicated cases.

The consultation paper emphasises its belief in the need for a culture of lifelong learning by health professionals. Continuing Professional Development (CPD) is defined as a process of lifelong learning for all individuals and teams which meets the needs of patients and delivers the health outcomes and healthcare priorities of the NHS and which enables professionals to expend and fulfil their potential. Whilst nursing as a profession has accepted CPD as a normal component of the job, medicine (especially with regards to consultants) has been less formal, leaving it largely to the individual.

The requirements of the Royal Colleges for Continuing Medical Education have evolved in the last 5 years and their impact on practice has yet to be evaluated. It is envisaged that links will be improved between CPD programmes, audit, clinical effectiveness and R&D and that all grades of staff will be expected to take advantage of these opportunities. The lifelong learning approach will also apply to the 400,000 non-qualified staff in the NHS, such as healthcare support workers and porters, etc. This is a challenging agenda for any healthcare organisation.

Commission to review at regular intervals

The overall role of the Commission for Health Improvement will no doubt develop during the next few years, but it seems likely that NHS Trusts will be subject to a review by the Commission at regular intervals. The implementation of National Service Frameworks (initially related to coronary heart disease and mental health), the recommendations of NICE, evidence of risk and complaint management and change of practice resulting from these, will be some of the areas covered by the Commission's visit. In addition National Performance Frameworks will monitor six areas of healthcare delivery, namely evidence of health improvement of populations, fair access to care, effective and efficient practice, patient or carer experience and finally outcomes.

The quotation from Yeats at the beginning of this introduction continues 'All changed, changed utterly: a terrible beauty is born'. The introduction of clinical governance has been broadly welcomed and the reasons for it understood; indeed to many it was incomprehensible that the Chief Executive was not, until now, responsible for the quality of care. It would be unfortunate, however, if the 'terrible beauty' of surveillance and bureaucracy believed to be needed to bring about this revolution is ultimately counter productive in terms of doctors' commitment and internal motivation[5], with increased costs and time not spent on direct care of patients.

References

1   Smith R. *All changed, changed utterly*. BMJ 1998; 316: 1917–1918.
2   The Stationery Office Ltd. 1997 *The new NHS. Modern. Dependable*. London: The Stationery Office, 1997.
3   *Bolitho* v *City and Hackney Health Authority* [1998] 9 Med LR 29.
4   Department of Health. *A first class service. Quality in the new NHS*. Health Services Circular 1998/113; 1998.
5   Smith R. *Regulation of doctors and the Bristol inquiry*. BMJ 1998; 317: 1539–1540.

▶2

Patient Expectations of Clinical Governance

Marianne Rigge

One of the most welcome statements in the government's quality consultation paper, *A first class service*, must surely be 'We need to move away from merely counting numbers . . . clinical governance will help ensure that quality resumes its rightful place at the heart of the NHS'[1].

Perhaps the biggest gap in the document however was a failure to define quality. If this is to be at the heart of the new concept of clinical governance, what is it likely to mean to patients, their carers and their representatives?

Openness and accountability

A starting point is to look at what happens when things go wrong in the dealings people have with the health service. Most of the research into the handling of complaints suggests that they want an explanation of what went wrong and why. They want to know who was responsible and they want to know what is going to be done to ensure that the same thing doesn't happen to someone else in the future. In other words, they want openness and accountability.

Much that is now being written about clinical governance centres around the formal systems that have been developed to stop problems occurring and improve the quality of care. Clinical audit, risk management, critical incident reporting, quality assurance, total quality management and so on are all part of this but the terms themselves would probably all sound quite alien to the average patient in the GP's surgery or on the hospital ward. This is because the health service has not so far been very good at explaining or reporting back in an open and accountable way on what these quality mechanisms are or what has been achieved as a result of adopting them.

As anyone who has ever made a formal, or indeed informal, complaint will know, the attitude they come up against is all too often one of defensiveness, prevarication, failure to explain or produce documentation that might help to do so, or explanations that seek to place the blame elsewhere – lack of staff, money, time or whatever.

Monitoring and evaluation

Part of the problem is that each of the activities mentioned above tend to be regarded as discrete, the responsibility of one person or team who may not be very senior, and almost certainly won't be accountable to the Chief Executive or Board. What is needed is a cultural change so that everyone working within the health service is signed up to the idea of quality being an intrinsic part of what they do all day and every day. Quality is about doing the right things at the right time and doing them right first time. It is about being able to identify the fact that something has gone wrong as soon as it has happened. It is about asking why, and then doing something about it. It is about setting up systems to enable this to happen, building in a continuing process of monitoring and evaluation and expecting to report back on the results of all this on a regular basis.

The rest of this chapter will explore some of the dimensions associated with quality from the patient's point of view. They are rarely articulated, not least because they are rarely asked for. Unless we pay greater heed to this, the term 'clinical governance' will remain as arcane and abstruse as 'clinical audit' has been to the millions of patients who have unwittingly taken part in it over the last decade or so at the cost of many millions of pounds which have not really been accounted for – certainly not in terms of results.

Looking back over what has happened to the NHS over that period, it is difficult to imagine how anyone allowed the introduction of that singularly ghastly statistic, the Finished Consultant Episode, or FCE, which allowed Ministers and others to boast that more patients than ever before were being treated. Nor have we yet escaped the obsession with counting. The record numbers of people on hospital waiting lists continue to be used as a political football, even though they are a totally inaccurate reflection of what is actually happening to those unfortunate enough to find themselves such a statistic.

Worst aspect of FCE system

The single worst aspect of the FCE system was that the 'F' in no way stood for 'finished' in any decent sense of the word. It might mean that some poor patient had been handed over to another consultant because the first, or even second, had been unable to reach a diagnosis. Or it might mean that a woman with breast cancer was first 'finished' by the surgeon she was 'under', then by the radiologist, then by the oncologist, possibly – after all that – literally finishing up under the palliative care specialist.

If we are truly interested in quality, it is high time that we stopped talking about people as 'episodes' or 'cases' and instead looked at the experience of patients as a whole. If we still need jargon – and the NHS seems positively to thrive on it – then 'patient pathway' or 'patient journey' would perhaps be a more appropriate definition of what we are trying to measure in our new all-embracing approach to quality.

I have long since tired of pointing out how inadequate is a system in which we record merely whether people were discharged or died as though it doesn't much matter which way up they leave the hospital. Under the current system, it is too easy to assume that as long as discharge takes place, the outcome must have been successful. The trend towards ever earlier discharge and much more day surgery is in most ways to be welcomed, but the lack of subsequent feedback to the hospital system from either patient or GP exacerbates a problem Florence Nightingale tackled far more successfully by recording whether or not patients were 'relieved' on their discharge.

Mortality statistics

Our current obsession with statistics extends to the way we treat death. In recent years, pressure has been building for the publication of mortality statistics so that we can compare hospitals' and surgeons' death rates. I admit to being part of this since I believe that the publication of data is itself a stimulus to improve the quality of that data, as well as to encourage informed debate about the reasons for variations, especially those that are unacceptable.

What we have singularly failed to do, however, is to devise ways of measuring the quality of the one certain outcome we all have to face – death. For many of us, the quality of care we receive from the NHS will be one of the most crucial factors in the quality of the manner of our dying.

Society has changed dramatically in the way it deals with death and the second most natural event in all our lives is nowadays more likely to take place in hospital than at home. And yet the quality of care at the time of death in hospital has been poorly researched and palliative care is not at the top of the audit agenda in most acute hospitals.

The Russian poet, Yevgeny Yevtushenko expressed far better than I ever could, just how important it is that we do not allow ourselves to depersonalise death by making it a statistic:

> No people are uninteresting . . .
> In any man who dies there dies with him
> His first snow and kiss and fight.
> It goes with him . . .
> Not people die but worlds die in them.[2]

The last time I quoted that poem in a speech was at the Royal College of Physicians' College Day on 11 July 1996 the day on which Anthony Hopkins tragically died. He had been in the audience and a member of his staff later asked me to send her the full poem because he had been so struck by it at the time. I was greatly moved when it was read out at his memorial service since it was clear from what his friends and colleagues said about him that he had managed to combine the scientific rigour with which he headed the RCP's research and audit department, with an extraordinary compassion and care for individual patients – to the extent that he publicly questioned the way in which clinical guideline development was heading, in a way I thought was very brave and much admired.[3]

Promotion of patient-centred care

My qualifications for contributing this chapter on patient expectations of clinical governance are those of a reasonably well-informed lay observer of the development of clinical audit over the past 15 years, during which I have been director of an organisation dedicated to the promotion of patient-centred care, the College of Health.

During some of this time, I was one of two lay members of the Clinical Outcomes Group, jointly chaired by the Chief Medical Officer and the Chief Nursing Officer. They have both demonstrated an unswerving commitment to the genuine involvement of patients and their representatives in every aspect of audit and quality control in all its manifestations.

But over the same period I have also served as a lone – and sometimes lonely – consumer representative on steering committees set up by medical Royal Colleges to produce guidelines for good practice in the treatment of cancer and other life-threatening diseases. I have been struck time and again by the overwhelmingly clinical approach to the production of guidelines – with an over-emphasis on hospital treatment – to the extent that some have almost wilfully refused to include appropriate referral or discharge criteria. I doubt I will ever forget a meeting at Richmond House, the headquarters of the Department of Health, at which a distinguished consultant said that the very idea of involving patients in audit was ridiculous and that the only person who could judge whether or not a hip replacement had been successful was the orthopaedic consultant who carried it out.

Qualitative research techniques

Since 1983, the College of Health has developed a range of qualitative research techniques to find out about patients' and carers' views and experience of the services they receive, which we call Consumer Audit.[4]

I hope to demonstrate that it is possible to add a vital extra dimension to clinical audit, risk management, quality assurance and clinical effectiveness as well as staff and organisational development – in short the basic ingredients of clinical governance – by involving patients and their representatives in all these activities. What is important is that the methods or techniques used to do this circumvent the typical barriers to genuine patient feedback. These are a combination of gratitude – 'the doctors and nurses were so wonderful but so overworked'; vulnerability – 'Well, you wouldn't really dare say anything when you know you might have to go back any time', or a deeply ingrained sense of knowing that whatever you might secretly think, 'doctor knows best'.

What we have shown in over 50 studies is that the people best placed to tell you about the most important dimensions of care – access, process and outcome, to use the jargon – are those at the receiving end, the patients.

Our studies have demonstrated, time and again, that it is not enough to look at one aspect of a service at a time through a series of uni-professional audits. By doing so, you will never discover that the vast majority of failures in the system are to do with poor communication, not just between doctors and patients, but between all the different health professionals and their colleagues in other disciplines. In our experience, most problems occur when patients fall through the net between their dealings with particular professionals.

Problems with access

A prime example is what happens to people during the time they are stuck on the hidden waiting lists before they are referred to a consultant. What most people don't realise is that it can be many years before the 'official' Patient's Charter target of 18 months starts ticking.

- **Case study.** Consumer audit of women undergoing elective hysterectomy

Although none of the women in this study had waited very long on the 'official' waiting list, many had in fact had the quality of their family, social, working and sex lives totally disrupted for up to ten years because of the failure of their GPs to take their problems seriously. 'He just said, "look, it's just part and parcel of being a woman, you've got to put up with it",' said one who had been reduced to wearing babies' nappies for her heavy periods.

Doing more harm than good

And it is only by asking patients about their actual experience that you discover that sometimes more harm than good is done during the long periods our system makes them wait.

- **Case study.** Long-wait orthopaedic patients

In a study of 50 patients before and after a hip or knee replacement, none was without pain and for some this had taken over their lives. 'The pain is just hell. I can think of nothing but pain. It's ruining my life.'

Some patients were taking up to and even over the maximum dosage of strong analgesics, including one man who had 'cut down' to 10 co-codamol a day because 'other drugs were doing terrible things to my insides over the years'. This was the same man who had spent so much money on an electric wheelchair, and a large van to put it in, that he could have had a private operation several times over. In the event, by the time he came to the head of the NHS queue, his joint had deteriorated so badly that he was left in as much pain and immobility as ever.

A number of patients in this study had to resort to non-drug methods of pain relief because of iatrogenic conditions such as ulcer or hiatus hernia, but the NHS did precious little to help. None was referred to a pain clinic and the one woman who had hydrotherapy on the NHS, which she found very helpful, was told that she'd had her limit after nine weeks – despite the fact that she still had another two years to wait. She had not been able to pay for more therapy privately because her condition had forced her to give up her job.

In both the consumer audits quoted above, our recommendations included the setting up of referral protocols between consultants and GPs and in the latter we suggested a multi-disciplinary protocol for the management and treatment of chronic pain.

We also suggested that social and financial factors ought to be taken into account when patients are prioritised for admission. Our evidence for this comes, not just from consumer audit research, but from more than 30,000 people who have been helped by the College of Health's National Waiting List Helpline.

The government's recent consultative document on the mechanism to replace extra contractual referrals (ECRs) unfortunately suggests that the current system enables GPs and patients to 'play the market' as though the exercise of informed choice were something wholly undesirable.[5] Yet time and again, patients tell us how they have been forced to spend their life savings or remortgage their homes in order to free themselves or their relatives from pain, preserve their sight or mobility, keep their jobs or carry on looking after a partner even frailer than themselves.

The following are real life case studies taken from our response to the consultative document on out of area treatment.[6]

● **Case study.** The effects on people's livelihood

An agricultural worker with two school-aged children had been on a very long waiting list for a knee operation. During this time his condition had deteriorated to such an extent that he was no longer able to work. Unfortunately, because he lived in a tied cottage, this meant that he would lose his home as well as his job.

● **Case study.** Life-threatening illness unsuspected

A woman had been waiting several months for a gynaecology out-patient appointment. Her GP thought she needed a prolapse repair. She was in considerable pain and discomfort and was concerned that the hospital could give her no idea when she could expect to be seen. We suggested a hospital in London where she could be seen and operated on within weeks. It turned out she had cancer and a hysterectomy was needed. She said if she hadn't rung the Helpline, she might still have been waiting, not knowing that her condition was life-threatening.

● **Case study.** GP's need for advice

One GP rang for advice following a health authority's refusal of an ECR for a patient with a complicated and long-standing leg ulcer when she acquired an antibiotic-resistant infection following a routine operation. The GP had arranged for community nurses to visit the patient daily but the ulcer was still failing to heal after many months. The GP had done some research and found a professor at a teaching hospital who is an expert in such cases. She pointed out that the cost of the nursing and the messing about that had been involved in complaining about the refused ECR must be costing the health authority much more than the cost of an out-patient referral to the teaching hospital, but she was chiefly concerned for the quality of her patient's life.

The last case study illustrates a fundamental failing in the way the current system works, especially in view of the fact that openness and accountability must surely lie at the heart of clinical governance. The proposed restriction on patients seeking treatment from specialists outside their district flies in the face of the government's attempts to modernise the delivery of health care by encouraging more informed decision-making.

Heightened public awareness

This is particularly the case at a time of heightened public awareness of unacceptable variations in mortality and morbidity, following the General Medical Council enquiry into the deaths of children undergoing heart surgery at the Bristol Royal Infirmary. At the same time it is being widely reported that more than half of all cancer patients are not being referred to an appropriate cancer specialist despite the Calman-Hine recommendations and an awareness that the UK performs poorly in the international league tables of cancer death rates.

The College of Health has a long-standing concern about the lack of information to patients on consultants' qualifications, training and special interests. This is particularly noticeable in the case of general surgeons and cancer. Our National Waiting List Helpline's most recent survey of acute trust waiting times, for first out-patient appointments and subsequent admission, specifically asked for information about consultants' special interests. An analysis of the first 125 responses showed that fewer than half the trusts were able to supply this information – and that was to GPs, never mind patients despite what it says in the Code of Practice on Openness in the NHS.[7]

With waiting lists only just beginning to drop from an all-time high, it does not make sense to impose new limits on the referral of patients from over-stretched hospitals to those which have spare capacity, especially when this could be paid for with the new funds being made available to reduce waiting lists.

It is difficult to see how primary care groups will be able to play a major part in ironing out inefficiencies and inequalities in the system if they do not have easy access to information about waiting lists and times, alongside appropriate performance indicator and outcome information.

The government's vision of a uniformly excellent NHS is greatly to be welcomed but even the Secretary of State admits that this may take ten years. Patients should surely not be denied the possibility of informed choice in the meantime.

The role of NICE

One of the most important functions of the new National Institute for Clinical Excellence (NICE) will be 'to produce and disseminate clinical guidelines based on relevant evidence of clinical and cost effectiveness and associated clinical audit methodologies and information on good practice'.[1] Consumer groups such as the College of Health have welcomed the announcement that membership of NICE will include patient interests, not least because of our experience in witnessing the development of clinical guidelines which have ignored the views of ordinary patients. The all-too easily accepted wisdom is that the gold standard for the production of guidelines is evidence from randomised controlled trials.

Next in the hierarchy comes evidence from systematic reviews of the scientific literature, followed by consensus statements produced by clinical experts. The experience and views of patients comes a clearly lagging fourth.

What many people do not realise is that randomised controlled trials tend to exclude certain rather important groups of patients, such as women of childbearing age, children, elderly people, people from ethnic minorities and those with co-morbidities, because they might spoil the science. Then there is the recognised bias towards reporting the results only of those trials which have been successful. In real life, most patients probably do not present with evidence-based illnesses and most professionals probably learn more from their failures than they do from their successes.

Medicine is an art as well as a science

A rigid insistence that guidelines must only be based on the evidence of scientific trials is unhelpful to patients. Medicine is an art as well as a science and sometimes results will depend as much on patient compliance as on the treatment administered. This, in turn, may depend on the quality of communication with patients and the information they are given.

One very welcome development has been the setting up of the Standing Advisory Group on Consumer Involvement in the NHS Research and Development Programme. This is a unique initiative with its own budget, support staff and freedom to commission research. Its first conference was oversubscribed and attended by 400 people from local and national organisations across the country as well as visitors from Australia and the Netherlands (both of which have government-funded national patient forums).

John Swales, Director of Research and Development at the Department of Health spoke eloquently at that conference about the importance of 'pragmatic trials' which evaluate the impact of treatment in the setting where it is delivered. 'The pragmatic trial is inseparable from evidence-based care. Its development has led us to recognise the essential part played by patients and carers'.[8]

His views were reiterated by the then minister, Baroness Jay, who said 'The argument goes far wider – we must also involve users across the range of health care, and those working in the NHS must accept users as partners in their own care and treatment, and involve them in decisions and choices.'

Involving patients in decisions and choices

The following two case studies are taken from consumer audits of breast cancer services carried out by the College of Health. They illustrate the right and wrong way of going about involving patients in decisions and choices.

● **Case study.**

'The doctor who did the test said, "Don't worry, I'm almost certain it's harmless". He really gave me false hopes. Then when I saw the consultant it was said very matter of fact, quite bluntly – "You've got cancer," he read from the report, "and you're going to have an operation". Then he turned and went out the door. That was the only really bad thing. I wanted to sit down and talk to somebody there and then. I think there is a very real need for some form of counselling. There I was left in this cubicle to get dressed and go home. You shouldn't simply be left to go home.'

It will come as no surprise that the recommendations of that consumer audit included training in counselling and communication skills for all staff caring for women with breast cancer and access to a breast care nurse during diagnosis and treatment.

The second study demonstrates a much better outcome for the surgeon concerned.

● Case study.

'I can't speak highly enough of the doctor. He was very gentle and kind and didn't hurry even though it was a busy clinic. He let me get dressed, then he sat me down and asked what I thought was wrong. When I said 'cancer', he said that was right but I shouldn't worry too much as the lump was small. When he'd let that sink in a bit, he asked me if I knew about all the different treatments and the pros and cons. He asked me if I'd understood and whether I had anyone outside to take me home or if there was someone the nurse could phone for me. He told me there was no hurry and that he wanted me to go home and think about what treatment I wanted and come back next week to talk again. He gave me the number of a nurse counsellor and asked me to get in touch with her if I was worried or I hadn't understood. It might seem funny, but I went out feeling really comforted and confident.'

Barriers to user involvement

Some of the barriers to user involvement in research and audit have been set out by Marcia Kelson, a senior research fellow at the College of Health who worked for a number of years for the patient sub-group of the Clinical Outcomes Group.[9,10] These barriers include professional resistance – the 'What could patients possibly contribute?' attitude previously mentioned; concerns about confidentiality (of consultants rather than patients in this context) and how representative or otherwise lay members, especially patients, can be expected to be. From the consumer perspective, there have been strong concerns about tokenism, about the lack of training and support and about a failure to recognise that people's time and willingness to be involved can be exploited, and that being involved costs money.[9,10,11,12]

Patient-defined outcomes

Another report by Marcia Kelson, prepared for the recently formed Effectiveness and Quality in Practice (EQUIP) group has highlighted the importance of patient-defined outcomes.[11] That work has since been built upon by the College of Health which was commissioned by the Royal College of Physicians with funding from the NHS Executive, to produce patient-centred guidelines for Rheumatoid Arthritis (RA) and Rehabilitation after Stroke. In both cases, focus groups of patients and carers were held around the country with the help of the key patient organisations. This method was deliberately chosen so that patients could talk about their experiences on their own terms.

In the past, clinical guidelines have tended to focus on issues that are important to clinicians and researchers, with an emphasis on test results and drug treatments. While there was discussion of these by patients in the focus groups, a considerable proportion of the discussions focussed on the impact of having had a stroke or having RA. Participants themselves observed that doctors tended to focus on clinical approaches while what was often needed just as much was advice on other services and sources of information and support. Many of the problems faced by both groups of patients have both emotional and practical consequences and can affect all aspects of their lives and relationships. It became clear that a holistic approach is needed and that this needs to involve health and social service professionals across the boundaries of primary, acute, community and social care.

With guidance from NICE, the development of such holistic partnerships, alongside the greater openness and accountability that clinical governance should bring in its wake, should help to secure recognised standards of care for patients, while maintaining necessary flexibility to accommodate different patient circumstances and preferences. However, if patients are to be encouraged, in partnership with clinicians, to make informed choices about their care and are to be assured that they are receiving the best standards of care available they, as much as health professionals, need access to the information contained in clinical guidelines. We need to ensure that information contained within the professional version of clinical guidelines is made available to patients in a patient-friendly format.

Clearly, there are cost implications attached to this, but if we are to have a truly quality-driven service such as that envisaged in *A first class service*,[1] then we must involve patients as active partners, and indeed experts, in their own health care, rather than the passive recipients we have expected them to be in the past. If clinical governance is to be a reality, they deserve no less.

References

1   Department of Health, *A First Class Service: Quality in the new NHS*, 1998.
2   Yevtushenko Y, *Selected poems, Penguin Modern European Poets*, 1962.
3   Hopkins A, Some reservations about clinical guidelines, *Archives of Disease in Childhood*, 1994, 72: 70–75.
4   College of Health, *Consumer Audit Guidelines*, London, 1994.
5   Department of Health, *The New NHS: Guidance on out of area treatment*, 1998.
6   College of Health, Response to the NHS consultative paper, *The New NHS: Guidance on out of area treatment*, 1998.
7   NHS Executive, *Code of Practice on Openness in the NHS*, 1995.
8   Consumer Involvement in the NHS Research and Development Programme, Research: what's in it for me? *Conference Report*, London, 1998.
9   Kelson M, User Involvement: a practical guide to developing effective user involvement strategies in the NHS, College of Health, 1997.
10 Kelson M, Consumer Involvement in the audit activities of the Royal Colleges and other professional bodies, College of Health, 1996.
11 Kelson M, Promoting patient involvement in clinical audit, Practical guidance on achieving effective involvement, College of Health, Clinical Outcomes Group Patient Subgroup, 1998.
12 Kelson M, Patient-Defined Outcomes, College of Health (in press) 1998.

▶3

Organisational Framework for Clinical Governance

Myriam Lugon, Jonathan Secker-Walker

The White Paper, when enacted, will place a new responsibility upon Trust Chief Executives. Until now an annual financial report had to be signed by the Chief Executive and agreed by the Trust Board, which guaranteed probity in the handling of public money by the Trust. A new requirement to sign a similar guarantee in relation to the quality of clinical care is the driving force behind the clinical governance initiative.

To be able to sign the annual clinical quality report, the Chief Executive will need to be assured that he or she is provided with regular information and performance indicators relating to the complex clinical environment.

Prior to the Conservative government's market reforms, hospital clinical organisational structure revolved around the 'Cogwheel' concept, with Divisions representing each specialty – or group of specialties. Chairmen of each Division met regularly as members of the Medical Executive Committee, the Chairman of which was usually the medical member of – or medical adviser to – the District Management Board or Team. There were usually several quality related committees that each reported to an individual Divisional Committee but which actually spanned horizontally across the District. Examples would be Infection Control, Blood Transfusion, Medical Records, Drugs and Therapeutics, Radiation Protection, Theatre Users and all of these committees would have their important recommendations taken to the Executive Committee and then onwards to the District Management Team.

In many new Trusts, Directorates replaced the cogwheel system, administrative assistance to the committees was cut to save money and in most cases, these committees did not die but had no support and no formal structure to which to report. Hence for the last half-decade many have functioned in a relative vacuum and have often not been as effective as they might have been.

Changes during the 1990s

The changes during the beginning of the 1990s included the introduction of clinical audit, the loss of Crown Immunity from prosecution for health and safety failure and the introduction of Crown Indemnity for NHS doctors. These all brought new quality committees into being; audit, risk management, health and safety requirements and latterly a new interest in the management of legal claims.

It is probable, therefore, that the medical director, when considering the complexity of introducing clinical governance, already has available a considerable quantity of existing information and expertise about the quality of care. To a degree the framework for governance will involve a structure that ensures that these quality committees make regular reports and are properly serviced so that minutes show responsibilities for action and clear recommendations.

The ideas explored in this chapter are personal to the authors. Clinical governance is such a new concept that there is no 'right' way to manage it and each Trust will adapt to fit its own circumstances and a national consensus will be arrived at by trial and error over a period of time. This chapter describes the organisational infrastructure required to deliver this agenda, the individuals/teams responsibilities and the place of quality in performance management.

Organisational infrastructure

The Trust Board and the Chief Executive need to be confident that clinical quality is monitored and that they are provided with regular reports to be warned of problems or deficiencies, in much the same way that monthly financial reports are scrutinised. It will be important for the Trust Board and Chief Executive to discuss and decide the nature of the information that they will require on a regular basis.

Monitoring of clinical quality depends on a standard against which to measure. It is often the case that Trusts have no formal mechanism for setting Trust-wide clinical policy. Individual directorates may work to guidelines – for instance the treatment of asthma in general medicine – but often these guidelines fail to cross directorate boundaries when orthopaedic or mental health patients happen to suffer from asthma for instance. The guidelines that are likely to be produced by the National Institute for Clinical Excellence will need to be formally accepted (or rejected if there are particular reasons), adopted and publicised by Trusts to form Trust protocols.

There is probably, therefore, sense in dividing the clinical governance structure into two distinct components; those of clinical *policy setting* and of clinical *policy monitoring* (Fig. 3.1). The engines that deliver these might be called the clinical policy committee and the clinical governance committee. Both should report to the Trust Executive Group that, in turn, would report to the Trust Board. The Trust Board may decide to extend the complaints and litigation sub-committee that often exists to include clinical governance or establish a separate clinical governance sub-committee (in some trusts this is the 'clinical standards' committee). The board sub-committee dealing with clinical governance would probably include the chief executive, a non-executive board member, the medical director and the director of nursing and would receive the minutes of the clinical governance committee.

Clinical Policy Committee

This committee which is likely to consist of clinical directors might serve several functions:

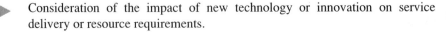 Be responsible for developing clinical strategy to promote clinical and financial viability in the future.

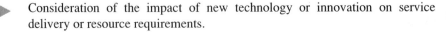 Consideration of the impact of new technology or innovation on service delivery or resource requirements.

▷ Adopting Trust-wide policy on clinical practice as a result of NICE, CEPOD, GMC, UKCC Calman/Hine, etc., or data from clinical governance committee and approving clinical protocols from directorates.

▷ Ensure implementation of R&D strategy.

▷ Assess benchmark data and recommend action with regard to changing clinical practice and improving value for money.

▷ Challenge the status quo of existing practice in the light of EBM or clinical effectiveness data.

Clinical Governance Committee

This committee would be responsible for gathering data from existing quality committees, risk management, complaints, claims and other information sources. It would be responsible for:

▷ Ensuring that standards of patient care are continuously improved in the light of the requirements of the Commission for Health Improvement, the GMC and the UKCC and other professional bodies.

▷ Providing advice to the Executive group, the Clinical Policy Committee and Directorates and influencing stakeholders both within the Trust and outside.

▷ Assigning responsibilities for the implementation of the Committee's recommendations to managers or directorates as appropriate.

▷ Monitoring the implementation of clinical governance and ensuring that recommendations from both the clinical policy and governance committees are properly disseminated and acted upon.

▷ Ensuring effective training and development of clinical staff.

▷ Developing effective and supportive measures for the management of poorly performing clinical colleagues.

▷ Facilitating the implementation of systems to underpin clinical governance; for instance, performance indicators, death rates, effective clinical audit, clinical incident data, complaints and claims data.

▷ Providing regular reports to the Executive and Trust Board and the Clinical Policy Committee.

The Membership of the Clinical Policy Committee needs to reflect the broad body of clinical staff. The Governance Committee is likely to include the clinician responsible for clinical audit, those responsible for risk, complaints and claims, and a university member where appropriate and the chairman of the medical staff committee or other 'unbiased' senior doctor. Some trusts are likely to involve a non-executive director in addition. The role of the Medical Director is crucial to both Committees but the chairmanship of the Policy Committee is clearly an essential component of the job. Leadership of the Governance Committee might well become the responsibility of a respected clinician or the Director of Nursing to whom, in some Trusts, many of the staff associated with quality monitoring jobs are managerially accountable.

At Executive and Board level both the clinical executive officers are members in any case and both groups would expect a consensus opinion to come from these two individuals.

The clinical governance committee (which could evolve from the clinical risk management committee) should receive the minutes – with recommendations where appropriate – from the following groups:

- ▶ infection control
- ▶ resuscitation
- ▶ medical records
- ▶ blood transfusion
- ▶ drug and therapeutics
- ▶ health and safety
- ▶ clinical audit
- ▶ clinical claims review
- ▶ radiation protection
- ▶ complaints and patient satisfaction
- ▶ pathology users
- ▶ theatre users.

Reports that impinge on the function of the Trust should be presented to the committee such as SAC reports on junior staff training, reports of Health and Safety Executive inspections, post-graduate deans visits and CPA accreditation visits to pathology laboratories.

The committee will require regular reports derived from performance indicators such as length of stay for specific operations or disease, deaths within 30 days of operation and treatments that are not considered to be effective – such as grommets in children or D&C in young women. A system needs to be put in place to capture this data proactively (e.g. a proforma to capture death rate information to be completed at the same time a death certificate is completed). Data should be available to staff by manipulation of the coded discharge summaries in the patient master index. This is often contracted out to a commercial IT company. This has the disadvantage of significant time lapse between the episode of care and seeing the data but the advantage of regular benchmarking against Trusts of a similar size and case-mix. An example of reporting infrastructure is shown in Figure 3.1.

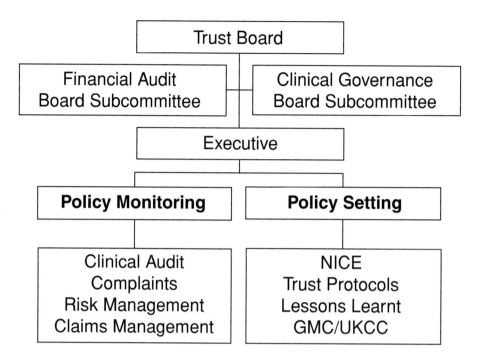

Fig. 3.1. Example of reporting infrastructure.

Delegated responsibilities

The Chief Executive is the officer accountable for the delivery of high standards of care. He/she, however, will need to identify the clinical lead to take the process forward within the organisation; this must be a Board level post – either the Medical Director or the Nursing Director. The lead will need to work very closely with his/her opposite number and with the Human Resources Director to ensure that clinical governance is included in an overall organisational development plan.

The lead will not only need to ensure that the reporting arrangements are clear and satisfy the Board that the appropriate processes are in place, but also investigate areas of concern and challenge clinical practice whenever necessary. The partnership between the Nursing Director and the Medical Director is critical if the delivery of this agenda is to succeed. The nursing profession has long accepted the concepts of working in teams according to clear guidelines and followed programmes of continuous professional development tailored to their individual and service needs; doctors (consultants) on the whole have been less formal about their practice and their personal and professional development – which has been largely left to an individual's decision.

We believe, therefore, that the Medical Director should be given the overall lead for the clinical governance initiative and that he/she should work closely with the Director of Nursing to ensure that explicit standards are set for clinical teams. We do not believe that organisations should consider giving joint lead to the two clinical members of the Board; this is likely to give confusing message to the organisation and may fragment the implementation process. The role of the Medical Director is described in detail in Chapter 12. Chief Executives should make clear to their organisation, however, that delivering high quality of care is everybody's responsibility both at an individual and team level and that performance management will include monitoring not only national performance indicators but also issues of clinical practice; this will be described later on in this chapter. The Chief Executive also needs to create the right environment for clinical quality to flourish; involving clinicians in management is one way to achieve this, as is the support of a team approach to reflective learning, currently adopted by nursing.

Role of the individual

Clinicians individually are responsible and accountable for their clinical practice; to this end they must ensure that they have the appropriate skills to deliver care safely and therefore ensure that their continuous professional development programme is aimed at the maintenance or acquisition of new skills if these are required. The trust will therefore need to establish a robust performance appraisal for all its staff (including the consultants) which will help identify the needs of individuals and services as far as continuous professional development is concerned. Individual clinicians must now monitor their own practice by taking part in clinical audit and by adhering to the policies and procedures of their organisations. They should also ensure that new techniques are introduced safely and by agreement. A framework for the introduction of new techniques is described in Chapter 8. Clinicians will also need to ensure that they fulfil the requirements for clinical supervision of junior members of staff.

Role of the clinical team

Care today is delivered in clinical teams usually centred on clinical directorates. In their document *Maintaining Good Medical Practice* published in July 1998, the General Medical Council acknowledges that care is delivered in a clinical team and that team members must demonstrate a commitment to effective clinical practice and good quality care and a willingness to learn.[1] The clinical team at a service level must ensure that clinical policies agreed at an organisational level are implemented; this may require the development of care pathways or guidelines. Where appropriate these should address the whole continuum of care from the GP practice, through the accident and emergency department or the outpatient clinic, to the inpatient stay and back to primary care. Services may therefore need to identify how they secure the advice and support of primary care for such development and thus address clinical governance issues across the interface. It may be appropriate for some conditions to include the steps taken in tertiary care and clarify the interface between primary, secondary and tertiary care. Addressing the whole continuum of care may require addressing social care needs for clients groups such as children, elderly, etc. This approach is likely to become more important as long term service agreements based on integrated care pathways, where appropriate, become the way services are commissioned.[2] Teams will also need to demonstrate that the care given meets the patients' needs and delivers good outcomes – although these are often difficult to quantify. To achieve this objective requires a process at service level to examine why untoward events, complaints and claims are occurring, identify trends and the action required to put things right; they should also monitor the implementation of national guidelines and health and safety issues.

Services, therefore, should set up multi-disciplinary clinical improvement groups[3] to receive their respective specialties' information on audit, risk management, claims and complaints. This group should be charged to identify any action required, training needs and link these to their training and education plan, to decide their audit priorities and consumer surveys requirements. An example of terms of references and composition of the group is given in Box 3.1 and is illustrated in Figure 3.2. The activity of the group should be open and transparent and thus be recorded. For issues crossing more than one specialty, the chair of the committee (often the clinical director) should be given the responsibility to negotiate with other directorates. Such

Box 3.1.	Clinical improvement groups
Membership	Multidisciplinary representation including nursing, doctors, paramedics; it should include both operational staff and directorate leads on clinical risk, clinical audit, education and complaints. The group should be chaired by the Clinical Director or their nominated deputy. It is supported by the clinical audit/risk department.
Objectives	▶ To review quality information, identifying potential problem areas and making recommendations to the Clinical Director. ▶ To co-ordinate clinical risk assessment in the directorate and oversee implementation of appropriate action. ▶ To ensure that all clinical areas are aware of potential risk to patients and staff. ▶ To review clinical incidents, claims and complaints in the directorate, identify trends and remedial action to be taken. ▶ To review customer satisfaction survey and identify service changes required. ▶ To make recommendation to the Clinical Director about actions to improve clinical practice and minimise risk such as development of standards/guidelines, development of care pathways, development of appropriate clinical policies and procedures. ▶ To identify appropriate training needs required to change practice and ensure that they are part of the directorate training programme. ▶ To be a forum where team performance can be monitored and where the clinical team development plan can be discussed.
Frequency of meeting	At least quarterly, more frequently if required.

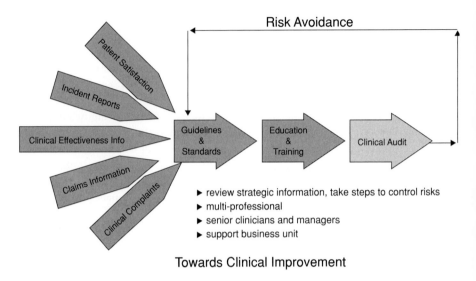

Fig. 3.2. Clinical improvement groups. Reproduced with permission from Burke C and Lugon M, © HRRI.

groups should be part of mainstream clinical business and could be used on a quarterly basis for performance monitoring purpose. Staff from clinical audit and risk departments should act as facilitators and change agents for these teams. The role of these groups in the process of managing claims is described in Chapter 8. The Clinical Governance Committee should consider the minutes of clinical improvement groups; the Clinical Governance Sub-committee of the Trust Board should monitor the delivery of the action plan.

Role of the managers

General Managers or Business Managers have so far found it difficult to intercede in matters of clinical practice; whilst it is not for them to dictate how patients are treated, they clearly have a role not only within the effectiveness field[4] but within the overall clinical governance agenda.[5] Indeed as Chief Executives are given statutory responsibility for the quality of care delivered, so too will managers need to understand their own responsibilities in ensuring that clinical practice is safe, and adheres to the relevant guidelines; where shortfall are identified they will need to support the team in taking the appropriate action. Managers must therefore foster a multidisciplinary approach to patients' care, an inquisitive culture where learning and reflecting on the team's and the individual's practice is part of the norm. They will need to ensure that the team adheres to the yearly individual performance review process necessary to identify training and education requirements and aggregate the individual plans at a team level to prepare a comprehensive and all inclusive training plan. In order to fulfil their role effectively, the managers will need to understand:

▶ how clinicians function

▶ how best practice is identified

▶ how practice can be monitored effectively

▶ what is meant by clinical risk management

▶ how complaints can be used to influence changes in clinical practice

▶ their own role within individual performance review.

This highlights the need for managers to receive the appropriate training and development to secure understanding of these processes. A partnership between clinicians and managers is necessary for the successful delivery of the quality agenda. Managers will need to facilitate and adopt a supportive approach, but may also need to challenge clinicians constructively. This identifies the significant cultural and organisational change required[6] and must be considered by the Chief Executive and the Human Resources Director as part of the trust organisational development agenda.

Role of the Board

Non Executive Directors have an important role to play in monitoring the quality of care provided by the various clinical services. To do this successfully they must have an understanding of the processes used for monitoring, such as clinical audit, clinical risk management, etc. Some training in these processes should probably be part of the development programme for Non Executive Directors, if they are to discharge their responsibility successfully. Non Executive Directors could be active participants of a Clinical Governance Committee and could be used as one of the drivers to ensure successful implementation of necessary changes in clinical practice. It is important that they feel able to challenge clinicians and managers in a constructive and non-threatening manner.

Monitoring performance

Quality reporting and monitoring should become a significant part of performance review. Many of the elements determining quality can be captured from clinical risk reporting, analysis of claims and the content of complaints. A template for quality reporting is described in Box 3.2. For most of these a trend analysis is necessary to determine whether the problem is one-off or recurring, the latter may warrant investigation and remedial action. A quarterly report is therefore most likely to be of use. This report should form part of the performance review of the various clinical services/ specialties; whenever necessary remedial action needs to be taken, the responsible individual and timescale for implementation needs to be identified and subsequently monitored. The manager of the service should be held accountable for the delivery of the action plan. It will also be necessary to include in the performance review process the national clinical indicators, performance framework information and other

Box 3.2. A template for quality reporting

Specialist Surgery

Clinical Claims

Business Unit/ Specialty	Total Cost	Trust Cost	New claims during Q2	Claims settled during Q2	Total number of Claims
Orthopaedics					
Ophthalmology					
ENT					
Total					

Clinical Incidents/Near Misses

Business Unit/ Specialty	Severity						
	Death	Severe	Moderate	Minor	Near miss	Not recorded	Totals
Orthopaedics							
Ophthalmology							
ENT							
Total							

Orthopaedic Incidents			
Event Type	Q4 97/98	Q1 98/99	Q2 98/99
Lack of Team Member			
Medication Errors			
Equipment Failure			
Other			

Clinical Complaints

Business Unit/ Specialty	Clinical Complaints Code (see Below)							Total
	1	2	3	4	5	6	7	
Orthopaedics								
Ophthalmology								
ENT								
Total								

contd.

Code	Description
CC1	Clinician failed to diagnose correctly.
CC2	Clinician failed to treat appropriately (no treatment or wrong treatment).
CC3	Clinician performed activities outside their competence/failed to seek guidance.
CC4	Clinician did not communicate adequately with patient/representative/guardian/ other clinical staff.
CC5	Clinician gave incorrect information to patient/representative/guardian.
CC6	Clinician had an abusive or dismissive attitude which upset the patient or failed to take into account patient or representative's sensitivities.
CC7	Other complaint of a clinical nature not covered by codes CC1–CC6.

Clinical Complaints			
Business Unit/Specialty	**Q4 97/98**	**Q1 98/99**	**Q2 98/99**
Orthopaedics			
Ophthalmology			
Oral Surgery			

Comments

measures of quality which trusts will be asked to report to the NHS Executive. It must, however, be recognised that systems and processes to monitor quality are unlikely to be at the same stage of development across all services in an organisation.

It is therefore necessary to audit in the first instance a baseline for services in order to identify which ones will need help and support from central function in order to progress. This audit should be simple and test not only the stage of development of each service with regard to the quality agenda but also test understanding of their responsibilities. An example of audit questions is given in Box 3.3. Monitoring development and progress in a large organisation can be complex. The authors therefore suggest that a system for self-assessment for clinical governance is developed based on the UK/European Model for Business Excellence;[7] this model is illustrated in Figure 3.3. This approach would have the benefits of involving staff in the process of continuous clinical improvements as well as empower and motivate them. Performance monitoring requires accurate and reliable data from quality indicators that are easily and repeatedly measurable.[8] There is much to be said for amalgamating staff in risk and claims management with complaints, audit, specialised IT and quality staff into central 'governance departments' and gradually developing generic governance workers related to and very familiar with each clinical department or group.

Box 3.3. Example of audit questions

Clinical Governance Survey

Q1 Directorate

Q2 Specialty

Director completing this form   Date: ....

This form should be completed fully and returned to the Risk Manager no later than .... (date).

Q3 Does the Service have individuals responsible for the management of the following:

	Yes	No
Clinical Risk Management	☐	☐
Clinical Audit	☐	☐
Complaints	☐	☐
Workforce planning	☐	☐
Co-ordination of clinical effectiveness information	☐	☐
Setting Service quality standards	☐	☐

Q4 Does the Service use the Trust Incident Reporting mechanism to ensure adverse events are identified?

Yes ☐
Sometimes ☐
Rarely ☐
No ☐

Q5 Are adverse events openly investigated, lessons learnt and changes made?

Yes ☐
Sometimes ☐
Rarely ☐
No ☐

Q6 Does the Service routinely assess clinical risks and put action plans in place to reduce risk to patients?

Yes ☐
No ☐

Q7 Is the quality of clinical record keeping (medical, nursing and other) routinely monitored?

Yes ☐
Sometimes ☐
Rarely ☐
No ☐

Q8 Does the Service have a clinical audit programme?

Yes ☐
No ☐

Q9 If Yes, does the programme involve all relevant clinical staff (medical, nursing, others)?

Yes ☐
No ☐

contd.

Q10 Do the results of audits bring about changes/improvements to working practices?
- Yes ☐
- Sometimes ☐
- Rarely ☐
- No ☐

Q11 Does the Service routinely hold a meeting to discuss quality issues, i.e. adverse incidents, complaints, clinical audit results, etc?
- Yes ☐
- No ☐

Q12 If Yes, what is the name of this meeting?

☐

Q13 Is this meeting multidisciplinary, involving all parties including managers?
- Yes ☐
- No ☐

Q14 Does this meeting recommend changes in how services are provided and ensure these happen?
- Yes ☐
- Sometimes ☐
- Rarely ☐
- No ☐

Q15 Are you discussing quality issues as part of the Service's business planning process?
- Yes ☐
- No ☐

Q16 Below are a number of statements, please rate how strongly you agree with each statement using the scale 1 to 5, where 1 = agree strongly, 5 = disagree strongly.

	1	2	3	4	5
Evidence based practice is supported and applied routinely in everyday practice.	☐	☐	☐	☐	☐
Workforce planning and development is fully integrated within the Service.	☐	☐	☐	☐	☐
Development programmes aimed at meeting the needs of individual health professionals and the Service needs are in place and supported locally.	☐	☐	☐	☐	☐
Processes for assuring the quality of clinical care are in place in the Service.	☐	☐	☐	☐	☐
Lessons are learnt from complaints and recurrence of similar problems avoided.	☐	☐	☐	☐	☐
Professional performance procedures that help an individual improve their performance are in place and understood by all staff.	☐	☐	☐	☐	☐
Clear procedures exist that allow staff to report concerns about a colleague's professional conduct and performance.	☐	☐	☐	☐	☐

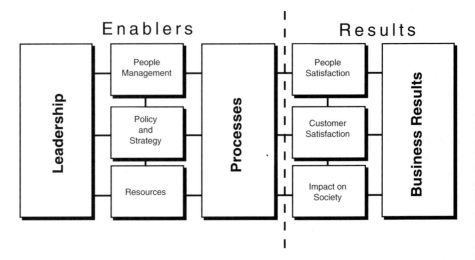

Fig. 3.3. The UK/European model. © British Quality Foundation (BQF) and European Foundation for Quality Management (EFQM).

Dealing with poor performance

Whilst it is recognised that the majority of staff working in the NHS strive to do their best for their patients, there are occasions – as the recent Bristol case has demonstrated – where the performance of doctors and other clinical staff is deficient. The Chief Medical Officer in his document *Maintaining Medical Excellence*[9] requires that healthcare organisations put in place procedures to identify and deal with performance issues early to prevent harm to patients. The British Association for Medical Managers translated this document into a procedure, which was disseminated to all Medical Directors. The authors suggest that this procedure be put in place in all trusts. The pathways for dealing with poor performance must be clear, explicit and widely disseminated and understood. As care is increasingly organised in clinical directorates, the authors suggest that the job description of Clinical Directors includes responsibility for dealing with poor performance and identifying remedial action. The emphasis, however, should be on prevention with identification of potential problems early.

The paper *Quality in the NHS. A first class service*[10] lists complaints, incident reporting, etc., as a way to monitor clinical performance and identify poorly performing staff. Such issues should be considered regularly by the clinical team to ensure that lessons are learnt and training provided where appropriate to avoid repeated untoward events and damage to patients. It is important that organisations are supportive of staff and invest in their training to avoid individuals operating at a level where they are no longer competent. However, if a serious shortfall in performance is identified through audit or clinical risk management, the individual clinician must be asked to stop the given intervention until he or she has received further training.

The BMA's Central Consultants and Specialists Advisory Committee[11] has recommended that Medical Directors set up a Professional Advisory Panel to investigate a problem at an early stage. It suggests that it is chaired by the chairman of the Medical Staff Committee, with the Clinical Director of the doctor concerned and a consultant from a neighbouring trust in the relevant specialty. The three wise men procedure may run in parallel where physical or mental health are thought to be involved. Any serious clinical incident should be investigated as described in Chapter 8. The organisation's approach should, however, be supportive and it should be ready to deal with problem doctors or nurses before patients are damaged but should ensure that the GMC/UKCC guidance is followed. In certain circumstances, however, the disciplinary procedure will need to be invoked. Such instances would include:

▶ Blatant disregard for the organisations' policies and procedures, or malicious or criminal intent.

Controls assurance

Organisations will need to pay attention to the relationship between clinical governance and controls assurance. Put simply, controls assurance requires the Directors of Trust Boards to satisfy themselves that systems are in place to ensure that risks are assessed and properly managed. To begin with the emphasis is on organisational and financial controls with such things as Standing Financial Instruction, Organisational Development Plans and Purchasing Strategies being regularly reviewed and updated. In due course this is expected to expand into other areas such as clinical risk and health and safety requirements.

Reporting to the Board

As mentioned earlier in this chapter, the Board will need to consider quality and clinical indicators on a regular basis; some information will be required monthly, some quarterly. It is important that the Chief Executive and the Trust Board agree the level of details required and the type of information provided. Information and data quality is dealt with in Chapter 13. It must also be recognised that information regarding clinical incident, claims and complaints will by definition deal with confidential data.

Whilst it is accepted that the NHS must be more open, putting some of this information into the public domain could damage patients' confidence and be threatening for staff. The format for the report will therefore need to be carefully considered. For example using the Audit Commission reporting format anonymising the data could be a way forward, a fictitious example is given in Table 3.1. It will also be necessary for each Trust to develop a good relationship with the local press highlighting the need to be supportive of the organisation's approach to quality.

Whilst the monitoring information should not be assigned to individual clinicians, the Board will want to adopt and/or develop clinical indicators by which services can

Table 3.1. Reporting and monitoring recommendations for serious clinical incidents – fictitious example.

Case No	Risk	Recommendations/control	Lead	Date	Completion
SCR001. 1	Misdiagnosis of acute pancreatitis and inappropriate management in A&E.	Include diagnosis and treatment in compulsory teaching sessions of A&E SHOs.	A&E consultant.	Oct. 99	
		Make all SHOs in A&E aware of the investigation results.	A&E consultant.	Aug. 99	Aug. 99
SCR001. 2	Traumatic effects of incidents on those involved.	Support individual doctor professionally and emotionally.	Consultant and senior nurse.	Aug. 99	Aug. 99
SCR002. 1	Risk of cross infection in theatres during eye surgery.	Review of aseptic practice within theatres.	Control of infection nurse.	Sep. 99	Sep. 99
		Implementation of recommendations from review.	Manager and consultant surgeon.	Nov. 99	
SCR002. 2	Availability of specialist opinion out of hours.	Circulate briefing note to all junior staff with contact out of hours for ophthalmology opinion.	Clinical Director ophthalmology.	Sep. 99	Sep. 99
SCR002. 3	Misdiagnosis of serious eye infection.	Include in training session for SHO in ophthalmology and A&E.	Clinical Director in ophthalmology.	Oct. 99	
SCR002. 4	Availability of medical records out of hours.	Improve process for accessing medical notes.	Patient's service manager.	Nov. 99	

be benchmarked against nationally available information. The difficulty in the use of indicators for monitoring healthcare quality has recently been discussed by Sheldon.[12] The implementation of the National Framework for Assessing Performance[13] will also lead to the production of comparative information. The Board will also need to ensure that they test services against the performance measures developed as part of National Service Frameworks. It will, however, be necessary to make explicit the quality standards that can be attained given the level of resources available locally.

Conclusion

Developing and implementing systems and processes to monitor clinical performance and the quality of clinical care needs time, effort, skills and resources. Much will depend on ease of access to good clinical information; an aspect of the NHS that in many Trusts is still woefully deficient. It is important that organisations recognise that clinical teams must be empowered to identify problems and deal with them, but also to be prepared to celebrate successes. The development of effective clinical team working is a necessary ingredient to the successful implementation of clinical governance as well as good change management processes. Clinical audit and risk staff as well as staff within complaints departments will need to work closely together providing their expertise to the clinical directorates thus facilitating changes in clinical and operational practice and help directorates deliver improved quality of care. This highlights a significant organisation and development agenda for any healthcare organisation. A clinical governance implementation plan must therefore be seen as part of an overall OD plan. To progress this agenda successfully, the Executive team will need to pool their effort to support this process and recognise that its success will depend on a steady evolution and not a revolution.

References

1   *Maintaining Good Medical Practice*. General Medical Council. July 1998.
2   HSC 98/198. *Commissioning in the new NHS*. Commissioning services 1999–2000. Department of Health.
3   Burke C and Lugon M. Integrating Clinical Risk and Audit – moving towards clinical governance. *The Health Risk Resource*. 1998 (2); 1: 16–18.
4   Dunning M, Lugon M and McDonald J. *Clinical Effectiveness. Is it a management issue?* BMJ 1998 316 (7127): 243–244.
5   Sutherland K and Dawson S. *Power and quality improvement in the new NHS: the role of doctors and managers*. Quality in Health Care 1998 (7) supplement: 16–23.
6   Donaldson LJ and Muir Gray JA. *Clinical governance: a quality duty for health organisations*. Quality in Health Care 1998 (7) supplement: 37–44.
7   UK/European Model for Business Excellence. British Quality Foundation (BQF) and European Foundation for Quality Management (EFQM) 1990–91.
8   Nelson EC, Splaine ME, Batalden PB and Plume SK. *Building Measurement and Data Collection into Medical Practice*. Annals of Internal Medicine. 1998; 128: 469–466.
9   *Maintaining Medical Excellence*. Chief Medical Officer 1995.
10   *Quality in the NHS. A First Class Service*. Department of Health. 1998.
11   Consultants issue guidance on professional advisory panels. BMJ 1998; 317: 1663.
12   Sheldon T. *Promoting health care quality: what role performance indicators?* Quality in Health Care 1998 (7) supplement: 45–50.
13   The Department of Health. *The new NHS. Modern. Dependable: A National Framework for Assessing Performance*. DOH 1998.

▶ 4
Integrated Care

David Hands

Introduction

The 1997/8 government White Papers[1,2,3,4] describe a *New NHS* committed to *'integrated care based on partnership and performance'*. Integrated Care is now the explicit basis for improvements in both efficiency and effectiveness. Improved effectiveness is the new focus of NHS performance, both in terms of improved treatment outcomes for individual patients and the promotion of population health.

Improved effectiveness is being promoted through a range of quality-orientated initiatives including Health Improvement Programmes, National Service Frameworks, Clinical Excellence and Evidence-Based Medicine. These initiatives will be supported by more clinically-focused information systems and outcome-orientated performance assessment. All parts of the Service are expected to embrace the concept of clinical governance *'so that quality is at the core of both their responsibilities as organisations and of each of their staff as individual professionals'*.

Performance judged on effectiveness is welcome to a service which has grown weary of previous inappropriate emphasis on crude measures of spurious efficiency such as numbers admitted to hospital. The purpose of the NHS is to improve population health and to make the sick healthier: its performance therefore needs to be assessed primarily by those yardsticks.

If integrated care is the foundation for improved effectiveness, it is important to understand what it means. This chapter, therefore, explores the concept of integration, the potential contribution of integrated care planning and management to the enhancement of clinical and organisational effectiveness and the relationship between integrated care and clinical governance.

The concept of integration

The dictionary defines integration as *'the combination of parts, or diverse elements, to make a whole.'*[5] This implies that, without integration, the intended object or process is imperfect. Conversely, *disintegration* implies the falling apart of something that is complete and effective for its purpose.

In industry, the connection between different companies that are engaged in successive stages of manufacturing is described as *vertical integration*. Collaboration or merger of firms that are engaged in the same kind of operation is called *lateral integration*. In psychology, integration is used to describe the reconciliation of the diverse elements of perception by combining different perspectives.

Integration, therefore, implies *the careful design and optimum combination of all of the diverse and necessary elements and perspectives of an activity in order to achieve the planned purpose and the best possible outcome.*

In health services, the integrative effort is primarily focused on individual patients who require an effective process of diagnosis and treatment to restore optimum health. However, because the health of individuals is a function of their environment and personal behaviour, the concept of integrated healthcare must also embrace the coordination of action to promote healthy environments and lifestyles. Integrated health planning and management must, therefore, cover the identification, analysis and solution of both individual and population health problems.

The dimensions of integration

Integration may be considered from various perspectives. Some of the most important are:

1. *Between component parts of the total system* (e.g. between the separate organisational entities which are responsible for prevention, primary, secondary, tertiary, continuing care and rehabilitation).
2. *Between different stages in the treatment process for a specific condition* (i.e. between initial tentative diagnosis through investigation, testing, final diagnosis, assessment, treatment and aftercare).
3. *Between different parts of the same service provider organisation* (e.g. the various parts of a hospital, such as clinical, diagnostic service, out patient, wards and hotel service departments).
4. *Between different health professions or between different specialties of the same profession* (e.g. between doctors, nurses and the professions allied to medicine).
5. *Between separate provider organisations of the same or similar kind* (e.g. between GP practices, hospitals or specialist service providers in different locations).
6. *Between the NHS and related organisations* (e.g. social services, housing, transport, environmental health and voluntary organisations).
7. *Between the commissioners and providers of services.*
8. *Between managers and clinicians.*
9. *Between different treatment or care regimes for different diseases or conditions in the same patient.*
10. *Between patients, their family, their home and social context.*

Integration of successive stages of a progressive process of treatment or care (types 1, 2 and possibly 3) might be described as *vertical. Lateral* integration involves coordinated working between everyone in the same field (types 3–10). Clearly each type is important in different ways to achieve maximum effectiveness from the patient's perspective. The challenge of integrated care is to ensure that each dimension is explicitly and systematically addressed, developed and designed in association with the others.

The barriers to integration

Despite the existence of a comprehensive NHS in the United Kingdom for over fifty years, many services can still be remarkably dis-integrated, even within an individual provider organisation. The progress of a patient between different parts of the overall system can be even more fragmented. Few services can demonstrate comprehensive and fully integrated care processes and structures which are *designed* systematically to achieve clearly identified target outcomes for each programme of prevention and treatment. Even fewer can validly show how outcome performance standards have been met or improved.

Despite the best of intentions, most clinical professionals know that treatment is not always delivered as well as it might be. Variations in access and outcomes are still excessive. Too often, incidents occur which show that clinical risk has not been minimised. Sometimes outcomes are out of tune with the real wishes of patients and their families. There is still considerable evidence of poor record-keeping and communications and time wasted on unplanned, duplicated or repeated activities.

It continues to be difficult to demonstrate the cost-effectiveness of treatment programmes. Whilst shortage, or poor allocation, of resources is undoubtedly an issue, continuing inefficiencies in the processes of care undermine the effectiveness of outcomes.

The reasons for this situation are complex. To a large extent, it has arisen because of the relatively haphazard way in which the NHS has evolved. In particular, the artificial *boundaries* which have grown around different NHS roles or institutions tend to impede patient-centred integration of the contributions to treatment and care.

The organisational structure of the NHS (e.g. the distinction between hospital and community based services) frequently creates boundaries which can impede continuity of care. Hospital organisation has traditionally been built around the skills of staff (e.g. medicine or surgery) rather than on patient conditions or needs (e.g. cancer services). In addition, inter-professional rivalry can impede effective teamwork.

The 1990 NHS Reforms fragmented healthcare providers and introduced a new boundary between commissioners and providers. The culture of competition impeded the development of cooperative networks although it probably encouraged a greater awareness of the patient as a customer.

There are also cultural factors which militate against implementation of systematic quality improvement techniques. These methodologies usually require standardised processes and audit of defined standards. Medical practice places emphasis on the personal clinical judgements of doctors and the uniqueness of individual patients. These values, whilst important, have encouraged the belief that any methodology which involves standardisation of treatment processes is either inappropriate or unworkable.

Finally, but not least, there are continuing rivalries between managers and clinicians. Health service management is still not as closely focused on quality for customers as in most other service organisations. Clinicians have also expected the quality of their skills and their good intentions to be taken for granted. The contracting culture has compelled both disciplines to begin to question previous assumptions. Clinical governance will accelerate that process.

Approaches to integration

Integrated planning and management of health promotion, prevention and clinical treatment requires the analysis and design, in classic Donabedian[6] style, of the structure and process of interventions required to produce the intended outcome. It also requires an understanding of the culture in which the society, the professions and services are set, the competencies or skills available and knowledge (evidence) about what is likely to be effective in specific circumstances.[7]

▶ *Vertical integration* requires careful design of the contribution of successive stages of the process of diagnosis and treatment. Attention must be given to management of the incidence and prevalence of a disease or condition in the community as well as the details of the treatment process for that condition when it arises in an individual. Care Pathways (see below) are likely to be useful if the treatment programme follows a relatively linear course.

▶ *Lateral integration* involves consideration of the contributions which might be made to prevention or treatment by the various health and health-related professions and by related services such as social services, voluntary organisations, housing or environmental health. This dimension is likely to be more important if the condition has multiple causes, is difficult to diagnose, or if treatment does not usually follow a straightforward linear process (for example, mental illness). It is also more relevant if the condition is chronic, complicated by other conditions or exacerbated by the environment in which the patient lives (such as in the elderly).

Several integrative approaches have already been developed in, or applied to, the NHS. The principal established contributions are:

The care group

Care groups were first introduced by the original 1974 NHS Planning System.[8] The system required plans for the development of services to be based on an analysis of the *needs* of specific groups of the population translated into the provision of the *skills* required to deal with the health problems in the *places* which were most appropriate.

This approach was relatively successful in relation to strategic planning services for groups such as children, the elderly, and the mentally ill. It was less successful in relation to acute, hospital-based services because the needs of such patients are so varied. Care group analysis is therefore a useful first step towards disease or condition-based planning.

Medical and clinical audit

Audit has formally been a feature of hospital medical practice since 1991.[9] Although it has been encouraged by the Department of Health and the medical Royal Colleges, it is still not strongly embedded as a routine in every hospital and specialty. Most audits have been retrospective studies of either aspects of treatment or unwanted outcomes. Medical audit has primarily been educational in orientation and has tended to be seen more as a component of learning and teaching than an element in the proactive design of better treatment processes.[10]

Audit in the General Medical Services is a more recent phenomenon but has been promoted with mixed success by Medical Audit Advisory Groups in each Health Authority area. Methodology has tended largely to mirror the retrospective approach of hospital practice.

Audit has also been practised throughout the NHS by the non-medical health and social care professions within their own areas of competence. Multidisciplinary clinical audit has been encouraged by the Department of Health[11] but has rarely been implemented systematically to secure continuous quality improvement (see below).

Continuous quality improvement

Continuous Quality Improvement (CQI) or *Total Quality Management* (TQM) methodologies have been very significant in improving the quality of many commercial products and services.[12,13] CQI/TQM is a philosophy which seeks to 'get it right first time' and achieve excellence in every aspect of customer service.[14] The development of this philosophy has been mainly driven by the consumer movement in the US and Europe where commercial success is increasingly dependent on quality rather than price.

The principal technique for applying CQI/TQM is 'systems re-engineering'. This involves rethinking the product or service from the customer's perspective and redesigning production processes to high standards to meet customer needs. CQI/TQM also requires a *Learning Organisation*.[15] Advocates of CQI/TQM in health care have recognised that the pursuit of quality is a continuing journey requiring humility and a willingness to learn from previous experience.[16,17]

The parameters of quality in healthcare were defined by Maxwell as Effectiveness, Efficiency, Equity, Accessibility, Acceptability, Appropriateness and Responsiveness.[18] These principles were the inspiration for many quality initiatives within the NHS. The Department of Health has encouraged these developments by dissemination of good practice and case studies.[19]

Local initiatives have involved various approaches such as quality circles and performance checklists. Some have incorporated external accreditation such as the King's Fund Accreditation Programme or the ISO 9000 series of quality assurance standards. The previous government's 'Patients' Charter' initiative also created several customer orientated standards. The Charter has recently been reviewed.[20] The NHS Executive also sponsored pilot systems-engineering projects at Leicester Royal Infirmary,[21] and elsewhere. Some of these projects have significantly improved efficiency and customer responsiveness.

These initiatives have helped the NHS to be more customer friendly but most have not addressed the more fundamental issue of clinical quality. It is rare for CQI/TQI initiatives to be integrated with clinical audit programmes or for clinical quality to be the driving force for process re-engineering. Many quality programmes have been effectively unidisciplinary (particularly in nursing), have tackled only the relatively superficial aspects of the service and have not found favour with many staff in direct contact with patients.[22]

Managed care

Managed Care originated in the USA where there is no universal healthcare system and where services are purchased and provided on the open market in a very wide variety of ways.[23,24] Most US patients are covered by one of many health insurance plans, often provided by employers. Historically, claims against these plans were made on a fee-for-service or per diem basis. However, the escalating cost of claims has caused the purchasers to become more proactive in managing their policyholder's treatment programmes and to negotiate inclusive packages for specific conditions with a network of preferred providers.

The original driving force was cost reduction but later methodologies have given more emphasis to quality. An important goal in the US context is to reduce over-consumption of unecessary or inappropriate treatment. Managed Care has therefore tended to emphasise primary and preventative care to promote wellness supported by efficient, adequate but not excessive, secondary and tertiary services. In a consumer-led society, the system has led to accusations that both clinical freedom and consumer choice are being restricted.

The value of US Managed Care experience to the United Kingdom is that the system has produced a plethora of clinical guidelines. Many are evidence-based and have been actuarially assessed and costed. Because they bring together most of the components required to produce reasonable outcomes at lowest cost and risk, these guidelines can be a useful starting point for developing Integrated Care Pathways (see below).

Disease management

Disease Management is also an American import which must therefore be assessed with knowledge of the context in which it evolved.[25,26,27] The purpose is to design a comprehensive, systematic approach to the treatment of a patient through the course of a condition or disease. Disease Management advocates pro-active, evidence-based case management and structured inter-professional/agency working. It usually involves active patient education and participation.

Disease Management has tended to work best with diseases about which most is known, for which it is easier to develop evidence-based protocols and where outcomes are more measurable. The approach has therefore been applied most frequently to chronic diseases of high incidence such as diabetes, heart disease, stroke, asthma, depression, substance misuse, AIDS and dermatological conditions.

Unfortunately, disease management has aroused some suspicions because of its association with American style cost containment. Concerns have also been expressed that the powerful focus on a single disease might conflict with a more holistic view of the patient. Furthermore, some pharmaceutical companies have been keen to develop the concept in partnership with clinicians. Whilst this might be helpful by supporting clinical practice with a pharmacological perspective, there have been concerns that this kind of relationship might bias treatment in favour of drug-based therapies and could encourage corruption. For these reasons the Department of Health initially prohibited commercial partnerships of this kind.[28] Later indications are that this hard line might be relaxed.[29]

Nevertheless, stripped of its commercial and transatlantic overtones, the underlying concept represents no more than structured commonsense in clinical practice. Its value lies in making explicit and pro-active that which has tended to remain implicit and re-active. The concept therefore offers the possibility of improving communications, testing assumptions and implementing real-time audit.

Risk management

The control of clinical risk is a crucial part of the quality jigsaw. The narrow view of risk management is that it is to protect the NHS from claims of negligence. The more positive view is that it is *a particular approach to improving the quality of care which places special emphasis on occasions in which patients are harmed or disturbed by their treatment*.[30]

Managed Care in the US was stimulated by the imperative for purchasers to control costs, but managing risk was equally crucial for providers. The exponential increase in litigation stimulated the development of risk control measures including sophisticated assessment methodologies, clinical indicators and care pathways. Litigation is now increasing in the UK and proactive risk management is being encouraged by the progressively more stringent standards promulgated by the NHS Litigation Authority.

Clinical risk management involves identification, analysis and control of risks by installing more explicit and standardised care processes and monitoring variances against defined parameters, usually within integrated care pathways (see below). The basic philosophy is therefore congruent with CQI/TQM and integrated care.

The Care Programme Approach (CPA)

The CPA was introduced in 1991[31,32] to improve lateral integration between the different professionals in health and social services who contribute to the care and treatment of people with mental health problems. The system was primarily intended to reduce the risk of patients causing harm to themselves and others.

Essentially, the CPA provides a structured framework and record system to assess and define treatment objectives and to monitor their achievement. Each patient is assigned a key worker who has specific responsibility for ensuring that all aspects of the patient's support are coordinated.

Evidence-based medicine

The White Papers make it clear that effective, integrated healthcare is to be grounded, as far as possible, on evidence-based medicine. The National Institute for Clinical

Excellence and the Commission for Health Improvement are intended to spearhead the identification and dissemination of best practice through National Service Frameworks. However, some of the groundwork has already been done.[33,34,35,36,37]

In 1991 the NHS Research and Development Strategy was launched with the aim 'to secure a knowledge-based health service in which clinical, managerial and policy decisions are based on sound and pertinent information'.[38] In 1992 the Cochrane Centre was founded as part of an international network committed to preparing, maintaining and disseminating systematic reviews of research on the effects of healthcare. Bulletins on *Effective Healthcare* were also initiated.

In 1993, the first official guidance on improving clinical effectiveness was issued by the Department of Health[39] and the health technology assessment programme was established. The NHS Centre for Reviews and Dissemination was created to provide information on the effectiveness of treatments and the delivery and organisation of health-care. The monthly journal, *Bandolier* began to be published by the Anglia and Oxford Region for the NHS R&D programme to provide regular updates on effectiveness. This followed an earlier initiative in that region to *Get Research into Practice* (GRIP).[40] A similar project, *Framework for Appropriate Care* (FACTS) was initiated in Sheffield.[41] These initiatives were pursued by the King's Fund in its project, *Promoting Action on Clinical Effectiveness* (PACE).[42]

In 1995, the journal *Evidence-based Medicine* was founded to provide reports on rigorously conducted new research drawn from a range of other journals. In 1996, the NHS Executive issued *Promoting Clinical Effectiveness*.[43] This framework built on previous experience of clinical audit and proposed a programme of sustained improvement throughout the NHS based on better information, innovation, and change management. The programme was later supplemented by a publication on *Clinical Guidelines*[44] and, in 1997, by a new, more outcome orientated framework for performance management[45] in the Service.

Several initiatives have therefore been taken to identify and promulgate evidence-based medicine. However, a survey of NHS Trusts, carried out in 1997, showed that while Clinical Effectiveness had featured on the agenda for most NHS Boards, it was far from being a regular, formal part of board discussions.[46]

Integrated Care Pathways (ICP)

The ICP is one of the most promising clinical management tools for the design of both vertical and horizontal integrated care. ICPs have emerged from several sources, including Managed Care and Risk Management. ICPs are known by a variety of names, including Coordinated Care Pathways, Anticipated Recovery Pathways, Care Maps, Clinical Algorithms and Multidisciplinary Pathways of Care.

ICPs have been defined as

> task orientated care plans which detail essential steps in the care of patients with a specific clinical problem and describe the patient's expected clinical course.[47]

They offer a structured means of developing and implementing defined protocols and processes of treatment and care. They also facilitate identification of variances from expected outcomes and therefore enable continuous audit and quality improvement.[48]

ICPs are used extensively in the Managed Care environment of the USA. Enthusiasm for their use is gaining ground in the UK. A UK National Pathway User group has been established to share and promulgate experience. ICP development is likely to gain momentum in response to the requirements of National Service Frameworks and clinical governance.

According to Campbell et al,[49] ICPs have been published for over 45 conditions in the UK. This number is almost certainly an underestimate. The number published worldwide is growing rapidly.

Some of the most interesting applications, and the implementation methodology, have been described in books by Wilson,[50] Johnson,[51] and Johnson and Norris.[52] Most of the early experience was in the acute sector, particularly surgery, where stages of treatment and outcomes can more readily be defined. However, ICPs have also been applied in the treatment of chronic diseases, such as asthma and diabetes, where the approach is similar to disease management. ICPs are also relevant in mental health services where they can helpfully build more detail around the CPA.

The process orientation of ICPs emphasises vertical integration but much of the value of development is that it encourages multidisciplinary learning. Wilson particularly emphasises multidisciplinary pathways which can also involve the patient and family.[53]

ICPs usually require an integrated, goal-orientated patient record which is used by all of the disciplines which contribute to the programme and may be held by the patient. This can significantly improve interdisciplinary effectiveness and reduce risk.

Intersectoral collaboration and 'Shared Care'

Intersectoral collaboration has been promoted by the World Health Organisation (WHO) in recognition that curatively-orientated healthcare systems have limited impact on the positive health of populations. Positive health promotion requires multi-agency action in relation to the environment and individual behaviour.

The intersectoral promotion of health has been recognised in the global WHO targets for *Health for All*.[54] They are reflected to varying degrees by individual governments in programmes such as *Our Healthier Nation*.[55]

The case for intersectoral action to combat poverty and ill-health has recently been restated by the Acheson report[56] which reinforces the messages of Black,[57] some 20 years earlier. Other proposals have also been made earlier for a coordinated national health strategy.[58] The present government has given renewed attention to positive health promotion by the appointment of a Minister for Public Health and the publication of Green Papers.[59] These envisage closer collaboration between health and local authorities to develop local Health Improvement Programmes. A programme of Health Action Zones,[60] focused on more deprived parts of the country, has also been initiated.

The consultative paper, *Partnership in Action*[61] and the White Paper *Modernising Social Services*[62] reinforce the need for closer lateral integration between health and local social services, particularly in relation to the community care of children, the elderly the disabled, and people with a learning disability or mental illness. For the first time a single, integrated inspection system for care and nursing homes is proposed.

Collaboration between health and social care has long been a policy of successive governments. In practice, it requires sustained attention to collaborative structures and practices at both individual, client and strategic management levels between all of the local statutory and voluntary agencies and local community groups. Studies have underlined the importance of a patient/client centred approach focused on quality and designed to build trust between the collaborating parties.

However, as noted earlier, boundaries continue to exist within the NHS. There have been significant recent shifts in the boundary between primary and secondary care. Specialist care is no longer synonymous with hospital care. Many specialist services (such as diabetes services, care of children and the elderly and psychiatry) have moved into a community setting. Many specialist procedures are now provided on a day-case basis including over 50% of surgery. The terms *Intermediate Care* or, preferably, *Shared Care* have been used to describe the new or changed settings in which specialist services can now be provided.

Pritchard and Hughes[64] have defined *shared care* as applying when

> the responsibility for the healthcare of the patient is shared between individuals or teams who are part of separate organisations, or where substantial organisational boundaries exist.

Their 1995 book records and analyses the reasons for success in a wide variety of initiatives including chronic illness, maternity services, investigation and diagnosis, emergency services, rehabilitation, terminal and palliative care and health promotion.

Organisational structure

An organisation's structure is most effective when it reflects the organisation's purpose: form should follow function. Whilst structures cannot guarantee appropriate outcomes, a poor structure can impede them. Structure is important because it reflects the distribution of accountability for different aspects of patient care: it needs to be carefully designed to support care and treatment processes.[65]

Organisation structures are rapidly evolving in the NHS. For example, hospitals are now frequently organised in 'Directorates' representing groupings of specific specialist skills. Some may be defined traditionally (such as 'surgery') but increasingly, directorates are beginning to reflect a more patient or disease-centred approach (such as 'oncology') which may provide a better foundation for integrated care.

Similarly, primary care organisation is moving progressively into larger units. The basic unit for the organisation of services is shifting from the District of 250,000 population to the 100,000 represented by the Primary Care Group/Trust. These changing structures need to be considered carefully and designed to reflect the distinctive contribution which each component is expected to make to the overall care of each kind of patient.

Certain individuals have a key integrative role in the structure. The most obvious is the General Practitioner who has continuing responsibility to integrate the overall treatment and care of individual patients.

The leadership role of consultant specialists is also important in relation to programmes of care for specific conditions. This is clearly evident in relation to services for children, the mentally ill or the elderly, and in relation to chronic disorders such as diabetes, heart disease, and asthma, where specialists are likely to have continuing responsibilities for patients over a longer time period

Some conditions, particularly chronic and degenerative disorders, justify the appointment of Case Managers who maintain regular contact with patients and ensure that care is progressing according to plan. Examples include specialist diabetes or palliative care nurses, health visitors and mental health key workers.

Managers also have key integrative responsibilities at all levels of the service. It is crucial that they work closely with clinicians to establish the governing frameworks within which integrated care can develop. This needs to include all aspects of patient-focused organisational development including research, training, and design of processes, structure and information systems.

Information systems

NHS information systems are slowly evolving to reflect the requirements of integrated care. NHS systems have traditionally been based on the administrative separation of 'Family Practitioner' and 'Hospital and Community' services. Likewise, within hospitals, separate systems have evolved for different functions, departments and disciplines.

Integrated information systems are an essential support to integrated care. It is vital that systems are designed upwards from clinical requirements. Management information needs can be met by aggregating data from individuals but never vice-versa.

The new national information strategy,[66] with its emphasis on individual patient identifiers and primacy of clinical information needs, shows more promise in supporting integrated care than its predecessors. New information systems need to be developed to support defined patient care processes, linking data about individual patients, with quality, outcomes, activity and resource use and to support the requirements for clinical governance[67] and Controls Assurance.[68]

Designing integrated care

The foregoing analysis of approaches to integrated care shows that the NHS already has experience of many of the key components. However, the impact of earlier initiatives has been fragmented. Future development requires integration and development of the best of earlier approaches.

The key stages of development of an integrated care programme may therefore best be described by synthesising the experience which has been gained from different approaches. This is summarised in the following eight steps. These are described in sequence but, in practice, the development path is more likely to be iterative than linear:

1. Problem identification

The first stage is to be clear about the focus for action. This will usually be the disease or condition for which integrated care is to be planned. If maximum impact is to be achieved, it is helpful to select a condition of high incidence or prevalence (e.g. heart disease, cancer or depression), one with large treatment volumes (e.g. hip replacement), of high risk to patients (e.g. childbirth) or high cost (e.g. transplant surgery). It is important to establish the parameters of the chosen condition with some precision (e.g. a specific type of cancer) and the basic facts about its relative incidence and prevalence in the local population.

2. Identification of key stakeholders

It is essential that the development programme should fire the imagination of everyone whose commitment is crucial to success. It is therefore crucial to spend time identifying and involving the key stakeholders who have an interest and a contribution to make, particularly those professionals whose established practice may need to change as a result of the analysis. As Pritchard and Hughes put it, there must be 'shared understanding of the domain from all viewpoints'.[69]

The participants will certainly need to include patient groups and those who might have an influence on prevention of the condition, such as local authority representatives from housing, transport or environmental health. The development group may also require representatives from any relevant industry and, possibly, representatives from research or commercial interests such as the pharmaceutical industry. At this stage it will be useful to identify a steering group for the project and the resources required to support it.

3. Identification of the knowledge base

The available knowledge about a condition and the evidence about its prevention and treatment must be gathered and shared by all concerned. This may involve a search in the literature or international databases. It is important to promote an environment of mutual learning and sharing.

An analysis of the impact of the current services, and their organisation and resource consumption will need to be undertaken so that a comparison can be made between the current arrangements and that which evidence suggests might be ideal. Frequently, there will be knowledge gaps. Here it will be important to be explicit about the assumptions which are being made. It may be necessary to commission research.

4. Establishment of targets and standards

Establishing realistic and measurable standards and targets is a difficult but essential part of the development process. Local discussion and development is essential to reaching better mutual understanding of different perspectives.

Published standards, guidelines and protocols are a good starting point but it is crucial that these should be critically reviewed and adjusted to suit local circumstances. Standards may relate to inputs, process or outcomes but as far as possible, outcome, or intermediate outcome, targets should be identified. It will be helpful to think through connections between the various measures and consider data collection methods. This will be important in relation to the information systems which will be required for monitoring and audit.

5. Re-engineering of treatment and care processes

A comparison of the map of current activities in relation to relevant evidence about best practice will invariably raise questions about whether current programmes are optimum. Some changes may be obvious and relatively easy to make but others might involve wholesale reconsideration of roles and responsibilities.

At this stage it is particularly helpful to consider the development of ICPs or use of disease-management methodologies. Some conditions require the identification of several pathway options or algorithms which depend on the variety of intermediate outcomes which may result from successive stages of intervention. ICPs should ideally cover the entire spectrum of the care process across organisational and professional boundaries.

Model pathways, programmes and record systems may be obtained from user groups, professional publications, or Managed Care guidelines. It helps to use an established pathway development tool and an experienced facilitator.

6. Redesign of organisation structures

The organisational structure may need adjustment to ensure that it is in the optimum configuration to support improved processes. It may be necessary to change the membership and responsiblities of the therapeutic team or the directorate structure. Specialist integrative or liaison roles may need to be created. It may be necessary to consider reshaping the structure on a care programme basis with associated information systems and budgets. There may be a need for reconfiguration of the boundaries of related organisations, staff transfers, joint appointments or secondments.

7. Redesign of audit, record and information systems

The redesign of care processes and structures must be accompanied by changes in record and information systems to ensure that treatment programmes can be continuously audited and reviewed. Most ICPs involve the use of an integrated treatment record in which target outcomes can be specified and the contribution of each profession recorded. It may be helpful for the patient to be the guardian of this record, particularly when the patient must play an active part in the programme.

Data collection and information systems must also reflect the changed processes and structures to enable real-time multidisciplinary clinical audit. This will probably entail the use of clinical decision support systems and pathway monitoring software.

8. Implementation and review

The development of an integrated care programme spanning the entire spectrum of care is likely to be a time-consuming project. It may be necessary to focus on one part of the total care spectrum at a time. Although, theoretically, it is logical to start with prevention, earlier success may be more achievable at another stage. If new pathways, treatment methods or information systems are being introduced it is of course always sensible to pilot them and progressively adjust their use in the light of experience.

Conclusion

The challenge of integrated care is considerable but one to which the NHS was always intended to respond. The Service already has within it the experience and commitment to promote yet more effective treatment and care. However, it has not always used that experience in a systematic and consistent manner across the full spectrum of care and has not always blended the significant insights which can be gained from the best of evidence-based clinical and management practice.

The collaborative agenda for *The New NHS* is probably the most exciting yet for those in the Service who wish genuinely to promote the improved effectiveness of patient care and improvements in population health. However, tackling that agenda will require leadership, enthusiasm, integrity and a willingness to learn. The NHS Executive publication, *A first class service*,[70] offers, for the first time, a framework for integrating all of the key aspects of quality by developing a programme focused on the six areas of:

▶ health improvement

▶ fair access to services

▶ effective delivery of appropriate healthcare

▶ efficiency

▶ patient and carer experience

▶ health outcomes of healthcare.

Governance involves establishing and continuously renewing the understanding of the purpose for which the organisation was established and developing the means by which that purpose might be achieved. If the purpose of the NHS is to produce the best outcomes for individuals through integrated healthcare, both organisational and clinical governance must be directed to designing the frameworks, processes and structures which will enable that purpose to be realised.

References

1   Great Britain. Parliament. *The New NHS. Modern. Dependable.* Cm 3807. Department of Health. London. The Stationery Office. December 1997.
2   Great Britain. Parliament. *Designed to Care: Renewing the National Health Service in Scotland.* Cm 3811. The Scottish Office. Edinburgh. The Stationery Office. December 1997.
3   Great Britain. Parliament. *NHS Wales: Putting Patients First.* Cm 3841. The Welsh Office. Cardiff. The Stationery Office. 1997.

4   Great Britain. Parliament. *Fit For the Future: a Consultation Document on the Government's Proposals for the Future of the Health and Personal Social Services in Northern Ireland*. Belfast. Department of Health and Social Services of Northern Ireland. 1998. (Consultative Document)

5   Concise Oxford English Dictionary. Sixth Edition. Oxford. 1979.

6   Donabedian A. *Evaluating the Quality of Medical Care*. Millbank Memorial Fund Quarterly. 1966. 44, at pp. 166–206.

7   Griffiths RK. Personal Communication.

8   Department of Health and Social Security. *The NHS Planning System*. London. June 1976.

9   Department of Health. *Medical Audit*. (NHS Reforms Working Paper 6) London 1989.

10   Paton C and McBride A. *Medical and Clinical Audit: Towards Quality?* In Paton C. *Health Policy and Management: the Health Care Agenda in a British Political Context*. Chapman and Hall. London. 1996.

11   Department of Health. *The Evolution of Clinical Audit*. London. 1994.

12   Deming WE. *Quality, Productivity and Competitive Position*. Centre for Advanced Engineering Study. Massachusetts Institute of Technology. Cambridge MA. 1982.

13   Hutchins D. *Achieve Total Quality*. Director Books. Hemel Hempstead. 1991.

14   Peters TJ. and Waterman RH. *In Search of Excellence: Lessons From America's Best Run Companies*. Harper and Row. New York. 1982.

15   Garret B. *Learning to Lead*. Harper Collins. London. 1991.

16   Berwick D. *Continuous Quality Improvement: an Ideal in Healthcare*. New England Journal of Medicine. 1989. 320: 53–56.

17   Berwick DM, Enthoven A and Bunker JP. *Quality Management in the NHS: the Doctor's Role*. British Medical Journal. 304, at pp. 235–239.

18   Maxwell R. *Quality Assessment in Health*. British Medical Journal. Vol. 288. 12 May 1984. pp. 1470–1471.

19   Department of Health. NHS Management Executive. *The Quality Journey: a Guide to Total Quality Management in Health*. EL(93)16. February 1993.

20   Dyke G. *The New Patient's Charter: a Different Approach*. Department of Health. 1998.

21   Leicester Royal Infirmary NHS Trust. *Re-engineering the Healthcare Process: Achieving Results*. Leicester 1996.

22   McDonald P. *Re-examine the Quality*. Health Service Journal. 7 September 1995.

23   Fairfield G, Hunter DJ, Mechanic D and Flemming R. *Managed Care: Origins, Principles and Evolution*. British Medical Journal. 314: 21 June 1997. pp. 1823–1827.

24   Fairfield G, Hunter DJ, Mechanic D and Flemming R. *Managed Care: Implications of Managed Care for Health Systems, Clinicians and Patients*. British Medical Journal. 28 June 1997. 314: 1895–1897.

25   Fairfield D and Hunter DJ. *Disease Management*. British Medical Journal. 315: 5 July 1997. pp. 50–53.

26   Hunter D. *Disease Management: Panacea or Placebo?* The Health Service Journal. 1995 105 (5473) at pp. 22–24.

27   *Disease Management*. The Health Service Journal Health Management Guide. Glaxo Welcome Supplement Issue No 7. 106 (suppl. 7) 1996.

28   NHS Executive. *Commercial Approaches to the NHS Regarding Disease Management Packages*. Circular EL (94) 94. NHS Executive. Leeds. 1994.

29   NHS Executive. *Partnerships with Industry for Disease Management: General Approach*. Discussion Paper. Leeds. NHS Executive. 1996.

30   Vincent C (Ed). *Clinical Risk Management*. London. BMJ Publishing Group. 1995.

31   Department of Health. *The Care Programme Approach for People with a Mental Illness Referred to the Specialist Mental Health Services*. London. Circular HC(90)23/LASSL(90)11. 1990.

32   Department of Health. *Building Bridges: a Guide to Arrangements for Inter-Agency Working for the Care and Protection of Severely Mentally Ill People*. London. 1995.

33   Appleby J, Walshe K and Ham C. *Acting on the Evidence: a Review of Clinical Effectiveness: Sources of Information, Dissemination and Implementation*. National Association of Health Authorities and Trusts. Birmingham. 1995.

34   Walshe K and Ham C. *Who's Acting on the Evidence?* Health Service Journal. 3 April 1997. pp. 22–24.

35   Muir Gray JA. *Evidence-based Healthcare. How to Make Health Policy and Management Decisions*. Churchill Livingstone. 1997.

36   Sackett DL, Rosenberg WMC, Gray JAM, Haynes RB and Richardson WS. *Evidence-based Medicine: What it is and What it Isn't*. British Medical Journal. 1996; 312: 71–72.

37   *Evidence-based Decision-Making*. The Health Service Journal Health Management Guide. Glaxo Welcome Supplement No. 6. 1996.

38   Department of Health. *Department of Health Research and Development Strategy*. Circular EL(91)66. London. 1991.

39   Department of Health. *Improving Clinical Effectiveness*. Circular EL(93)115. London. 1993.

40   Dunning M, McQuay H and Milne R. *Getting a Grip.* Health Service Journal. 28 April 1994. pp. 24–26.

41   Eve R, Golton I, Munro J and Musson G. *Learning from Facts – Lessons from the Framework for Appropriate Care Throughout Sheffield (FACTS) Project.* ScHARR, University of Sheffield. Occasional Paper No. 97/3. Sheffield. May 1997.

42   Dunning M, Abi-Ahad G, Gilbert D, Gillam S and Livett H. *Turning Evidence into Everyday Practice.* King's Fund Publishing. London. 1998.

43   NHS Executive. *Promoting Clinical Effectiveness.* Leeds. NHS Executive. 1996.

44   NHS Executive. *Clinical Guidelines: Using Clinical Guidelines to Improve Patient Care Within the NHS.* NHS Executive. Leeds. May 1996.

45   NHS Executive. *The New NHS. Modern. Dependable: A National Framework for Assessing Performance.* Consultation document. NHS Executive. Leeds. January 1998.

46   Walshe K and Ham C. Op cit. 1997.

47   Campbell H, Hotchkiss R, Bradshaw N and Porteus M. *Integrated Care Pathways.* British Medical Journal. 316: 10 January 1998: 133–137.

48   Hands DM and Wilson J. *Integrated Care Management.* The Health Care Risk Resource. The Health Service Journal. 9 June 1997.

49   Campbell H et al. Op cit. 1998.

50   Wilson J (Ed). *Integrated Care Management: the Path to Success?* Oxford. Butterworth Heinemann. 1997.

51   Johnson S (Ed). *Pathways of Care.* Blackwell Science. Oxford. 1997.

52   Johnson S and Norris T. *Managing Integrated Care Pathways.* Blackwell Science. Oxford. 1998.

53   Wilson J. 1997. Op cit.

54   World Health Organisation. Regional Office in Europe. *Targets for Health for All: Targets in Support of the European Regional Strategy for Health for All.* WHO. Copenhagen. 1985.

55   Department of Health. *Our Healthier Nation.* Green Paper on the Future of Public Health in England. The Stationery Office. London. 1998.

56   Acheson R. *Independent Report into Inequalities in Health.* The Stationery Office. December 1998.

57   Townsend P and Davidson N (Eds). *Inequalities in Health: the Black Report.* Penguin Books. Harmondsworth. 1982.

58   Jacobson B, Smith A and Whitehead M. *The Nation's Health: a Report from an Independent Multidisciplinary Committee.* King Edward's Hospital Fund For London. London. 1991.

59   Department of Health. Op cit. 1998. Similar consultative documents have been produced for Scotland, Wales and Northern Ireland.

60   Department of Health. *Health Action Zones.* Circular EL(97)65/LASSL(97)21. London. October 1997.

61   Department of Health. *Partnership in Action.* London. 1998.

62   Great Britain. Parliament. *Modernising Social Services.* Department of Health. The Stationery Office. London. December 1998.

63   Smith R, Gaster L, Harrison L, Martin L, Means R and Thistlethwaite P. *Working Together for Better Community Care.* School for Advanced Urban Studies. The University of Bristol. Bristol. 1993.

64   Pritchard P and Hughes J. *Shared Care: the Future Imperative?* The Nuffield Provincial Hospitals Trust. Royal Society of Medicine Press. 1995.

65   Hands DM. *Evidence-based Organisation design: the Contribution of the Health Services Organisation Research Unit at Brunel University.* The Nuffield Trust. 1999.

66   NHS Executive. *Information for Health.* NHS Executive Report A1103. NHS Executive Leeds. September 1998.

67   Scally G and Donaldson LJ. *Clinical Governance and the Drive for Quality in the New NHS in England.* British Medical Journal. Vol. 317. 4 July 1998. pp. 61–65.

68   NHS Executive. *Corporate Governance in the NHS: Controls Assurance Statements.* Circular HSG (97) 17. NHS Executive. Leeds. March 1997.

69   Pritchard P and Hughes J. Op cit. p. 206.

70   NHS Executive. *A First Class Service: Quality in the New NHS.* NHS Executive. Leeds. 1998.

▶5

Clinical Effectiveness and Evidence Based Medicine: Some Implementation Issues

Ewan Ferlie

Introduction and background

Implementing EBM – a problem as well as a solution

A major component of the new corporate governance agenda is the assuring of evidence based medicine (EBM), or more broadly, evidence based practice. The last five years have seen increased policy level support for the principles of EBM and this may well continue in the future, but with the higher tiers of NHS Trusts being given more explicit responsibility for local implementation. The Medical Director and other Board members (for example, CEO, the Director of Nursing) will play a pivotal role in such quality assurance systems and may be audited on their performance. But in what sense, can they really 'implement' EBM within their organisations?

One's response depends on how one analyses the rise, nature and impact of the EBM movement. The underlying case for EBM is not new[1] and indeed who could be in favour of clinical practice not founded in evidence? The political and public opinion drive behind these reforms has been given impetus by a few high profile cases which suggest that existing systems of clinical self regulation were badly flawed. However, the widespread implementation of EBM over the last five years has been hindered by the lack of local clinical ownership as the EBM movement attracts at least as many critics as supporters. The result is that beyond a few bridgeheads, EBM may be proclaimed as corporate policy in theory; but also ignored in clinical practice. There are few reasons to suppose that this pattern will shift in the absence of a long term culture change or (more negatively) a high profile crisis.

What implications does this argument have for the design of clinical governance systems? This paper addresses this question from a social science perspective, in particular from the discipline of Organisation Behaviour (OB). It also draws on primary empirical data[2] collected by Wood, Ferlie and FitzGerald on the implementation of clinical research and speculates what these data imply for the worlds of policy and practice.

Securing change in professionalised organisations: some basic ideas

Decision makers operating in a complex environment (such as health care organisations) may find that a conceptual framework helps make sense of a mass of information and guides action. From an OB perspective, EBM ideas call for clinical practice – and eventually health care policy making – to be based on a data based and formal mode of rationality. This perspective is quite different from the political mode of rationality[3] previously dominant in health care policy or indeed concepts of tacit or implicit knowledge[4] where clinical practice is seen as much as a learned craft as a science.

While policy is made centrally; it is enacted locally within clinical groups. This raises the question of implementation and of implementation deficits which may well occur. A linear and rationalistic approach is often evident in the calls to 'implement' research into practice which are frequently made[5,6] by the policy system or in some academic writing. The power of the corporate core to do this is limited by the continuing autonomy of a range of professional groups. Professionalised organisations[7] represent a distinctive organisational form based on a collegial pattern of control and high levels of worker control over work practices. Clinicians typically build their own work roles rather than fit into present ones,[8] and new clinical groupings spontaneously emerge reflecting the growth of new fields. There is a norm of 'gentlemanly' (sic) conduct which results in a failure to tackle 'difficult' colleagues effectively. 'Real' practice resides at front line level, with the corporate core often having only marginal importance.[10] This clinical dominance rests on knowledge power as clinicians typically have more knowledge about their fields than their clients, health care purchasers or Board members. Clinical knowledge may include strong tacit elements, as professionals know more about their practice than they can say explicitly. Such knowledge is exchanged through informal professional networks, which may exclude non professionals. This tacit knowledge may be particular to a clinical specialty so that even a Medical Director would have difficulty in accessing it from outside.

The literature on change within autonomous professionalised organisations suggests a successful display[10] of change resistance from professional power groups when confronted by externally generated initiatives. A crude imposition of EBM principles may well lead to the defeat of the Board and of the Medical Director who would thus be placed in an untenable position. So clinical performance issues are best tackled by a body of part time clinical managers operating within their own fields, perhaps supported by business and general managers. The development of this cadre is complex and time consuming and health care organisations display marked variation in the capacity, commitment and enthusiasm of such cadres of clinical managers,[11] reflecting their histories and long term investment decisions over the last decade.

Study design and methods

This paper reports the findings of a recent study[2] designed to identify the scientific, organisational and behavioural factors associated with clinical behaviour change. We used a qualitative design, namely comparative case studies. Case studies are indicated where it is important to capture the meaning attributed to actions to explore informal processes which lie behind formal decisions. This is particularly helpful where there are different stakeholders, each advancing a different version of reality. The unit of analysis was the career of a clinical change issue and cases were selected so as to:

▶ make comparisons between those seen as strongly evidence based and those not so strongly evidence based. In making this assessment, we drew on already published work which highlighted possible candidates for evidence based medicine interventions and also took advice from an Advisory Group which included eminent clinicians and nurses. We wanted to assess whether those issues seen as evidence based diffused more rapidly than those that did not

▶ secure a spread across different clinical settings (e.g. medicine and surgery). We were interested to assess whether the pattern previously identified in surgery of highly volatile change[12] was still in place.

	Medical	Surgical
Favourable evaluative evidence	Decision support system for anticoagulation clinic (devolved from secondary to primary care)	Low molecular weight heparin (LMWH) in elective orthopaedic surgery
Less favourable evaluative evidence	'Changing Childbirth': issues of risk assessment	Minimal access surgery for inguinal hernia

Fig. 5.1.   Case study selection matrix.

Our research objectives were formally stated as follows:

▶ To study the career of four different change issues designed to secure change in clinical practice within the acute sector.

▶ To establish the relative uptake/impact of each change, identifying the scientific, organisational and behavioural factors which shaped these change outcomes.

The research was divided into two Stages. Stage 1 was an overview of the four issues across the sponsoring NHS region using a list of decision makers supplied by region and subsequent snowballing names. Each researcher led on a particular issue and in all 71 in depth interviews were undertaken. A semi structured interview schedule was developed which contained a common core section (needed for comparative analysis) and also an issue specific section. All 71 interviews lasted 1–2 hours, were fully transcribed and subjected to contents analysis. In addition, the team searched for written material including articles, guidelines, trial results and letters to clinical journals.

Stage 2 consisted of a further 48 in depth interviews within four sites selected for an intensive micro analysis (giving a total of 119 interviews). Such local groups were selected because they exemplified the change issues derived in Stage 1. A second interview schedule was developed and a customised version applied to all respondents. Secondary data included minutes of meetings and grey literature. Finally, informal observation was undertaken 'on site', supplemented by ad hoc discussions with 5 patients in one case. Respondents were selected after a period of observation because they were important in the decision making process. Respondents in the two stages were drawn from three key occupational groups: clinical consultants ($n = 52$), junior medical staff ($n = 9$) and nurses ($n = 23$). A few general managers ($n = 3$) were interviewed but only where they emerged as important.

Overall empirical results

For reasons of brevity, only the key thematic results across the case studies are outlined, here and their implications for policy and practice explored. The individual analyses are contained in Wood et al.[2]

> ▶ *Finding 1: There was no strong relationship found between the strength of the evidence base and the rate of adoption of the innovation.*

The push from the science base is only one factor in clinical decision making and just because there is strong scientific evidence to support a clinical innovation, does not mean that it is more rapidly adopted. In our study, the oral anticoagulation project received a very positive evaluation and was strongly 'evidence based', but still found it difficult to move forward, with budgetary issues and medico-legal implications needing to be settled before it could diffuse. It was not that the innovation was actively rejected – it was relatively uncontroversial compared to the other three – but high levels of indifference were enough to slow its spread.

The pro LMWH evidence suggested by a literature review which had been used to select this issue as 'evidence based' was heavily contested in the field. This confirms the argument that the 'world' of meta analysis remains divorced from the world of clinical practice,[13] and that knowledge may flow poorly between the two groups. Although orthopaedic practice was changing, there was no fixed trend towards LMWH but rather a pattern of volatility apparent, with some local groups adopting heparin or indeed other modalities but then retreating.

Minimal access surgery for inguinal hernia was founded in little primary data, at least in its early days. Nevertheless, practice change within surgery was rapid, if also contested and volatile. Different camps emerged, with different views on what constituted good practice given that there was a choice available. The 'Changing Childbirth' document was seen as more politically than scientifically led, and was the only case in which a sophisticated implementation strategy was apparent. Where local conditions were right, it was an effective lever for reshaping practice, although there were also some units where change was not so rapid.

The career of clinical innovations is thus strongly affected by organisational and behavioral factors as well as scientific evidence. Linear or 'stage like' models of implementation or diffusion are seriously misleading and the implementation process is far more interactive, negotiated and uncertain. These may be very general arguments: some Canadian evidence suggests[14] that the extensive development of clinical guidelines and protocols has had only limited effects on clinical practice. While an OB influenced literature highlights this lack of linearity,[15,16] this knowledge has not yet been reflected in the design of EBM implementation strategies!

Implications of finding 1 for policy and practice

NHS Boards now have responsibility for effective local implementation strategies to help assure evidence based practice. Our data suggest that a local implementation strategy may well be needed, as the push from science is by itself relatively weak. A range of factors can block clinical behaviour change (such as the incentives facing GPs; the number of organisational boundaries involved in the career of the innovation) or indeed promote it (role of professional opinion leaders; fear of litigation). Change is most likely to occur where all these sets of factors coincide, and an important appraisal task at Board level may well be to identify and intervene in these receptive settings for change.[17]

However, our data also indicate that linear and corporate wide models of implementation are seriously misleading and are likely to end in serious implementation deficits. We suggest that effective implementation strategies will be more localised, more negotiative and more interactive than assumed in the linear model. The corporate core of the organisation has a shaping role, influencing the key decisions which are largely made within clinical groups. So the core needs to be in frequent interaction with receptive clinical groups, resourcing and supporting bottom up energy for change. An important role is to select, resource and develop key clinical leaders who can manage change within their own groups.

▶ *Finding 2: Scientific evidence is in part a social construction as well as 'objective' data.*

Sometimes, the world of meta analyses paints a picture of science as a cool, formal and neutral activity. Here is science without scientists. But we cannot fully understand science without understanding how scientists produce and debate their science.[18] Science itself is validated by such essentially social processes as critical debate and controversy, refereeing and review procedures. Scientific knowledge is often highly provisional in nature and subject to radical revision as new data emerge. The idea that a consensus would emerge if only enough RCTs were conducted was naïve. In the orthopaedics case, the view from metaanalysis that the issue had been settled (in favour of LMWH) was contested in the field. Despite this attempt to impose a settlement on the controversy, debate reopened during the period of fieldwork with major researchers taking up opposite positions on an issue which was technical (the

Pulmonary Embolus event rate) but also had major implications for the validity of previously well received studies. Such controversies were evident within professional communities (e.g. the role of laparoscopic techniques within surgery) but also between them. For example, obstetricians and midwives were engaged in a debate about what actually constituted good evidence in relation to 'Changing Childbirth'.[19]

In most of these cases, there was no such entity as 'the body of evidence' but rather competing bodies of evidence available. Much of what is called evidence is in fact a contested domain, constructed from the debates and controversies produced by opposing viewpoints.[18] Even the construction of the research agenda itself and of perceived legitimate research methodologies is influenced by such contest. For example, should we always regard RCT based evidence as the most valid form of evidence or are there problems in which other forms of evidence are more appropriate?

We are certainly not taking a radically subjectivist line which argues that there is no such thing as evidence! Scientific controversies included technical debates (over the quality of research design or of data sets) as well as being influenced by backstage social factors. Rather we see clinical research as an arena where the natural and the social worlds intersect. But science is in part a social process, with a D phase as well as an R phase and thus scientists seek to enroll others into their projects (through the adoption of knowledge validating roles as editors, Research Directors, referees or expert advisers). The LMWH debate within the orthopaedics case would be a good exemplar of the operation of these social processes within science. An important role of the scientific investigator may well be to pay active attention to this *enrolment process*.[20]

Our data suggest that research may have more impact when it effectively combines with local forms of clinical knowledge. Failure of the research results to move into the world of GPs helped explain the stalled career of the anti-coagulation innovation. The pattern is also evident in the complaint of pro LMWH researchers operating outside the orthopaedic community about their inability to move the results from general surgery into orthopaedics. Scripting in national professional leaders was seen as a way of helping this translation process.

Implications of finding 2 for policy and practice

The scientific basis of many health care interventions remains contested, even by those clinicians who actively follow the evolution of the science. There may be relatively few areas where there is conclusive evidence, but many where there is continuing debate. The evidence base for a proposed intervention must be seen as convincing within the professional field concerned. Nothing could be more damaging to the EBM movement than to propose an intervention as 'evidence based' which was in fact not so. Nor are meta analyses based on RCT data[13] always accepted by practising clinicians, who often use a wider range of data sources.

This is not a counsel of despair, but it is an argument for subtlety. There may be a range of interventions within a particular field which can all claim some positive evidence, but also others which have none. Clinicians should *not* be using certain techniques, although it is not appropriate to insist on one particular intervention. While most clinicians within a group may be operating within acceptable professional opinion, others may be extreme outliers. It may be appropriate to ask for evidence that clinicians have updated their knowledge bases and have actively reflected on their practice, rather than that they come to a certain and universal solution.

There may also be sources of 'high impact' research which should be easier to implement locally. The literature on the diffusion of research suggests this will often be where there are long standing patterns of interpersonal interaction between researchers and end users of research.[21] Teaching hospitals and collaborating centres in multi-site trials might well offer receptive sites for the production of 'home grown' research results.

▶ *Finding 3: There are different forms of evidence differentially accepted by different individuals and occupational groups.*

To add to the complexity, there are perceived hierarchies of evidence, where the position in the hierarchy relates to the credibility of the source as well as the 'hardness' of the data. For some, RCT designs were the most credible, especially if results were published in highly reputable and widely read journals with tight peer review procedures. In our study different views of what constituted high quality research were encountered. Interestingly, perceptions of hierarchies of evidence are not stable between the different professional groups[19,22] which characterise many health care settings. Nor did these groups share many common journals or data sources, so research may flow very poorly across occupational boundaries. A specialist journal could be widely accepted by one professional subgroup, yet dismissed by others.

To what extent was the RCT seen as the 'gold standard' of research design? Within our data, many hospital consultants held up the RCT as 'the gold standard' in theory, although in practice some found ways of critiquing existing RCTs when they produced results with which they disagreed. Both surgical cases illustrated the strength of the RCT research paradigm, at least as an aspiration held by many (but not all consultants). Yet RCT results were also inconclusive and contested. There had been 25 years of RCTs in the orthopaedics case, yet it was still argued by some surgical practitioners that 'there was nothing out there'.

Other professional groups were less wedded to the RCT method and accepted alternative designs. Primary care workers may be more sceptical about the applicability of RCTs, with major problems around control groups. Midwifery respondents underlined limits to RCT based research, arguing that it does not look at the experience of the mother and the process of childbirth. For example, the amount of pain – as experienced by the mother – was seen as under researched because it was 'soft' and hard to quantify, but nevertheless a crucial measure of outcome. Midwives also argued that the views and choices of mothers needed to be incorporated into the research process and current research was described as over reliant on clinical assessment.

Some surgeons saw surgery as a craft rather than as a science, pointing out that techniques – even if backed by research – did not readily transfer from one unit to another. Rather surgical practitioners gradually accumulated tacit knowledge and craft skills, learning 'what worked for them' by reflecting on their results rather than displaying a total reliance on the results of RCTs.

Implications of finding 3 for policy and practice

Views about what counts as evidence are deeply engrained beliefs which are difficult to shift. The distrust of formal science by some practising clinicians has already been identified by Greer's[23] study of medical technology adoption decisions and is confirmed in this study. At a group level, the effective implementation of many research findings requires a range of different occupational groups to work together within multi-disciplinary settings. Yet each profession – or even specialty within a single profession – developed its own knowledge base, insulated from neighbouring knowledge bases. Nor were these blockages to the diffusion of knowledge being actively diagnosed or worked on in many of the sites in our study.

At a minimum, these blockages need to be actively surfaced and debated, perhaps using job plans, Continuing Professional Development, the audit machinery, or the Development arm of the R and D function (which may be crucial in linking the research base to practice change). Individual clinicians can be encouraged to reflect on the knowledge base which underpins their practice, how to update it, and to consider whether to amend their own learning style.

The intergroup issues also need to be addressed explicitly through the construction of linking bodies which bring the different groups involved in the implementation of research evidence together, preferably within a learning environment and outside the busy daily routine. The key question is: what is acceptable to whom as high quality research? These learning events may take the form of short courses designed for a mixed audience, a further degree course at a local University, or through an explicitly multi-disciplinary research or development group. This further reinforces the need for health care professionals to move out of traditional uni-professional contexts and to work effectively in multi-disciplinary settings where no one occupational group has dominance over the production of knowledge.

The ability to create a genuine learning environment in which these processes can occur may be a strategic priority for health care organisations as the link between a capacity for accelerated learning (which may take place at the level of the individual, the group or the organisation) and a capacity to manage change has been highlighted in the generic literature.[24]

> ### Finding 4: The data identify specific organisational and social factors which affect the career and outcome of clinical change issues.

Our data also identify specific organisational and social factors associated with a stronger or weaker flow of scientific knowledge. Knowledge flowed poorly across boundaries, whether organisational, occupational or knowledge boundaries. So innovations which involved antagonistic or multiple stakeholders (each of which could block change) faced particular difficulties. Each of the stakeholders will react according to the particular mix of incentives which they face. Some of the innovations involved the complex renegotiation of roles between a large range of clinical professions[26] rather than change within a single profession, and thus raised issues of professional jurisdiction. Often expert knowledge remained contained within localised professional communities of knowledge to which it was difficult for outsiders to secure access. Exceptionally, the 'Changing Childbirth' case suggested that the presence of a vocal Social Movement Organisation (e.g. the National Childbirth Trust) could reinforce political pressure for change on professionals, but this was a rare example of externally led change. It was also associated with a purpose designed implementation strategy which followed on from widespread consultation.

Professional networks remained resilient (despite general managers and internal markets) so that local clinical 'buy in' is essential in progressing change. Change which was purely driven from outside was unlikely to make headway within local clinical groups, where much discretion over working practices still resided. The case for change is enhanced by clinical product champions,[23,25] both nationally and locally. Such advocates can bring credibility and establish leadership within their professional groupings by their active support of an innovation. Science is more likely to diffuse when it can be effectively 'translated' into the world of local practitioners, many of whom use forms of knowledge which are craft based, tacit and experiential. A key variable in achieving change is the extent to which an initiative can achieve a 'fit' and be recognised and adopted within local frames of reference[20] and sponsorship by recognised professional leaders may help achieve this fit.

Implications of finding 4 for policy and practice

It may be possible to use external pressure (for example, from consumer of advocacy groups) to facilitate clinical behaviour change, in particular when such groups form effective alliances with health care staff. But the presence of clinical leadership for change remains a key factor as professional networks remain firmly embedded in decision making. Such leadership may come from national opinion leaders, professional networks or colleges.[26] However, our data suggest that local clinical groups are also important, and that their behaviour can vary substantially. Clinical groups which exhibited good interpersonal relations appeared to be more open to learning and change so that influencing the climate of such clinical groups may well be a strategic task. This may involve the spotting and developing of new clinical product champions, although it is important that these clinicians should be able to function as team players rather than individual 'stars' if they are to be able to persuade colleagues.

The 'Changing Childbirth' case also suggested that the presence of a well thought out and top led implementation strategy could accelerate practice change, at least where it coincided with a receptive climate at local level. So the most effective implementation strategies may combine top down pressure and bottom up energy, rather than being purely bottom up in nature. Such implementation strategies may well involve the diagnosis of organisational and behavioural forces which influence research implementation locally, for example, by changing the incentive mix facing a particular occupational group or by using preexisting pressure from professional colleges to remedy a local situation.

▶ *Finding 5: The upper tiers of the NHS, health care purchasers, R and D and the general management function generally played only a marginal role in the change process.*

The data suggested the continuing resilience of professional groups in shaping local work practices. The higher tiers of the health care system – including the R and D function, local NHS Boards and general management – were largely absent. Our data thus confirm the findings of Rosen and Mays[22] but suggest a more marginal role for the strategic or Board level tier of the organisation than argued by Greer[28] in American technology adoption decisions.

The possible exceptions were the anti-coagulation case but here the influence of the R and D function was tied to the provision of (time limited) funding and the 'Changing Childbirth' case, where there was a top down implementation strategy, but one devised after consultation with professional and other stakeholders. Even here, local 'bottom up' factors and willingness to embrace change was important and interacted with the top down push. There was little evidence within our cases of imposed clinical protocols, performance indicators, externally generated standards or care pathways, based on meta analyses or produced by outside experts. Our data suggest that the impact of such ideas on reshaping clinical practice may so far be relatively contained.

There was little evidence of health care purchasers – either Health Authorities or GP Fundholders – forcing clinical change through the contract, despite initial hopes that purchasers would provide a vehicle for practice change. Where they did (as in one 'Changing Childbirth' locale), there was some evidence that they were being driven by advocacy groups or Social Movement Organisations. Purchasers were not seen as possessing the technical knowledge required to question clinical practice credibly, and their expertise further diminished as health care purchasing organisations downsized , or went through a prolonged period of turbulence and reorganisation. They were focused on crude indicators of cost and activity. Primary care budget holders possessed even less R and D knowledge with which to question practice. Even in the politically visible 'Changing Childbirth' case which involved substantial investment decisions, the pressure for change from purchasers or NHS Boards was generally minimal.

Implication of finding 5 for policy and practice

The retention of professional control over most practice decisions is not an accident, but reflects continuing professional dominance and knowledge power. Previous reorganisations have made only very limited impact at this level; and unless the fundamental conditions change, it is difficult to see future reorganisations changing this picture.

 The present extent of professional dominance may be reduced in the future through increased litigation, radical consumerism and recourse to the courts, although this also depends on the behaviour of judges.

 Secondly, our data reinforce the need to embed change within the professions themselves through the development of effective professional leadership, including clinician managers who are prepared to tackle individual clinical performance issues where necessary.

▶ Thirdly, while existing systems of self regulation have proved grossly inadequate in some areas, and more effective measures need to be taken against extreme outliers, it is still important to develop more effective self regulation.

This may well be of a more transparent nature than hitherto and include a greater external and lay component in order to restore confidence.

Concluding discussion

The results of a small scale study are reported here, but they confirm the findings of other recent UK studies[13,22] into patterns of clinical behaviour change and the importance of local and often tacit clinical communities of practice. Taken as a whole, this research base suggests there may be limits to the rapid or broad implementation of EBM principles into practice.

▶ The policy system may need to pick EBM interventions with care, and avoid those where the evidence could be contested as such initiatives could quickly unravel.

▶ Secondly, implementation is more likely to succeed whether there is active professional support, especially the presence of a local clinical change agent.

▶ Thirdly, attention needs to be given to active boundary spanning and facilitation so that knowledge can flow across conventional boundaries.

There is now increasing recognition by clinical researchers of the gap between research evidence and actual clinical practice,[29] and an awareness that even simple changes to clinical practice sit in a complex organisational context. 'Implementation' is increasingly revealed as a key stage in the whole research cycle. Social science based research such as this can produce a body of knowledge which is potentially useful and available to help implementors as they strive to design clinical governance systems. In keeping with the spirit of the analysis, it is recognised that such research will represent only one factor in such design efforts but where local conditions are right, it may represent a powerful lever for system change.

References

1   Cochrane AL (1972) *Effectiveness and Efficiency: Random Reflections on Health Services.* London: The Nuffield Provincial Hospitals Trust.
2   Wood M, Ferlie E and FitzGerald L (1998) *Achieving Change in Clinical Practice: Scientific, Organisational and Behavioural Processes*, University of Warwick: Centre for Corporate Strategy and Change.
3   Alford R (1975) *Health Care Politics*, London: University of Chicago Press.
4   Polanyi M (1966) *The Tacit Dimension*, London: Routledge and Kegan Paul.
5   Department of Health (1991) *Research for Health*, London: HMSO.
6   Banta HD and Behney C (1981) 'Policy Formulation and Technology Assessment', *Milbank Memorial Quarterly*, 59, at pp. 445–479.
7   Montgomery K and Olivier A (1996) 'Responses by Professionalised Organisations to Multiple and Ambiguous Institutional Environments – The Case of AIDS', *Organisational Studies*, 17(4), at pp. 563–572.

8   Friedson, E (1994) *Professionalism Reborn*, Cambridge: Polity Press.
9   Bucher R and Stelling J (1969) 'Characteristics of Professional Organisations', *Journal of Health and Social Behaviour*, 10, at pp. 3–15.
10 Hinings C, Brown, JL and Greenwood R (1991) 'Change in an Autonomous Professional Organisation', *Journal of Management Studies*, 28(4), at pp. 375–394.
11 Ferlie E, Ashburner L, Fitzgerald L and Pettigrew A (1996) *The New Public Management in Action*, Oxford: Oxford University Press, Chapter 7.
12 Stocking B and Morrison SL (1978) *The Image and the Reality*, Oxford: Oxford University Press for Nuffield Provincial Hospitals Trust.
13 Dawson S (1997) 'Inhabiting Different Worlds – How Can Research Relate to Practice?', *Quality in Health Care*, 6(4), at pp. 1–2.
14 Rappolt SG (1997) 'Clinical Guidelines and the Fate of Medical Autonomy in Ontario', *Social Science and Medicine*, 44(7), at pp. 977–987.
15 Mulrow C (1996) 'Critical Look at Critical Guidelines', in Peckham, M. and Smith R. (eds) *Scientific Basis of Health Services*, London: BMJ Publishing.
16 Oxman A (1994) *No Magic Bullets: A Systematic Review of Interventions to Improve the Performance of Health Care*, London: North East Thames RHA.
17 Pettigrew A, Ferlie E and McKee L (1992) *Shaping Strategic Change*, London: Sage.
18 Latour B (1987) *Science in Action: How to Follow Scientists and Engineers Through Society*, Cambridge, Mass: Harvard University Press.
19 FitzGerald L, Ferlie E, Wood M and Hawkins C (1998) 'Evidence into Practice? An Exploratory Analysis of the Interpretation of Evidence', in (eds) Mark A and Dopson S *Organisational Behaviour Research in Health Care*, London: Macmillan, in press.
20 Wood M, Ferlie E and FitzGerald L (1998) 'Achieving Clinical Behaviour Change: A Case of Becoming Indeterminate', *Social Science and Medicine*, forthcoming.
21 Faulkner W and Sender J (1995) *Knowledge Frontiers*, Oxford: Oxford University Press.
22 Rosen R and Mays N (1998) 'The Impact of the UK NHS Purchaser Provider Split on the 'Rational' Introduction of New Medical Technologies', *Health Policy*, 43, at pp. 103–123.
23 Greer A (1988) 'The State of the Art Versus The State of the Science', *International Journal of Technology Assessment in Health Care*, 4, at pp. 5–26.
24 Pedler M, Burgoyne J and Boydell T (1991) *The Learning Company*, London: McGraw Hill.
25 Pettigrew A, Ferlie E and McKee L (1992) *Shaping Strategic Change*, London: Sage.
26 Abbott A (1988) *The System of Professions*, Chicago: University of Chicago Press.
27 Crane D (1972) *Invisible Colleges*, Chicago: University of Chicago Press.
28 Greer A (1984) 'Medical Technology and Professional Dominance Theory', *Social Science and Medicine*, 18(10), at pp. 809–817.
29 Haines A and Donald A (1998) 'Making Better Use of Research Findings', *British Medical Journal*, 317, at pp. 72–75.

▶6

Clinical Audit and Clinical Governance

Conor Burke, Myriam Lugon

Introduction

With the recent Publication of *A first class service*,[1] quality standards will become central to local health services. This represents a remarkable shift in health policy from a primary responsibility for financial performance, to a position where financial and quality performance are equally balanced and given the same priority. It follows that if quality standards are the central means of improving services, then the mechanism for monitoring and ensuring these are delivered, will undoubtedly be clinical audit.

Audit as a concept, has been used within Health Services since their first inception. A formal definition and responsibility for audit first came into being in the late 1980s with the advent of medical audit.[2] At this time the emphasis was on the importance of medical audit as a medically led initiative the purpose of audit being educational and not managerial. This was reinforced by many of the royal colleges who emphasised that the principle of audit discussions should remain confidential.[3] The next evolution in audit followed in 1993, when the integration of medical audit with nursing and therapy audit led to the term clinical audit and the advent of a multi-disciplinary approach. At this time audit was referred to as not just an educational process but as a real means for changing clinical practice and improving the quality of a service.[4]

Since this time the impact of audit has received a lot of attention and as a result there have been many critics[5] and fewer advocates[6] of the audit process. One of the consistent allegations made of clinical audit is its inability to change practice,[7] however, few texts or educational initiatives have ever addressed this most complex issue. Instead, much of audit seems to have focused on measuring activity, with little consideration about how to change or improve performance. Malby (1995)[8] suggests that change is the key link in the audit cycle and that audit should only be undertaken if the area to be reviewed can be changed. The future of quality in the NHS will undoubtedly depend on the ability of services to change, adapt and improve accordingly. This chapter considers a change model, relating it to audit and suggests a framework for integrating these within clinical governance.

Changing practice

Change in organisations happens all the time. It is often a subtle cumulative process that is accepted within normal operating activities. The consequences of uncontrolled change are impossible to predict and can be devastating and lead to chaos. To be successful, organisations must manage change in a pro-active and planned way that minimises risks, while accomplishing corporate goals. Clinical audit is designed as a structured cycle of change, where actions are taken following a review of existing practices. Actions are often based on educational initiatives that seek to achieve change in knowledge and clinical practice. However, according to Rogers (1983)[9] enabling change is not just about education. Having changed the knowledge base individuals need to analyse new information and form an opinion. Once an opinion has been formed the individual can decide whether to adopt or reject the change. Adopting the change will mean that they begin to implement this within their practice, testing its appropriateness. Finally for change to be effective the adoption of an innovation needs to be sustained and also adopted by the rest of the team or service within which the individual works. In effect, achieving change is about influencing attitudes, behaviour and organisational culture, as well as education.

One approach that attempts to address the whole of the change cycle within an operational setting is encapsulated within the Open Systems Model.[10] According to Beckhard et al (1993)[11] the open systems approach has four key steps:

 Identifying what is driving change, its power and the control you have over this.

 Describing how the future will be. This may involve setting goals or standards to be achieved.

Assessing the current situation or setting a baseline in comparison to future objectives.

Defining what is required to get from the present to the future, including the management of this process.

All of the above steps are not necessarily sequential but demand may require us to give each simultaneous attention in order to arrive at a solution. Beckhard et al (1993) have published a useful illustration of this process in their book *Organizational Transitions* (Fig. 6.1). The rest of the chapter discusses how the clinical audit process can produce effective and sustained changes in practice when used within an open systems model. The text gives examples of how clinical audit links with other governance initiatives such as risk management and continuing professional development.

Identifying the need for change

The nature of change forces

With the change in government health policy, a number of driving forces can be identified:

 the development of technology

new legislation

increased public expectations.

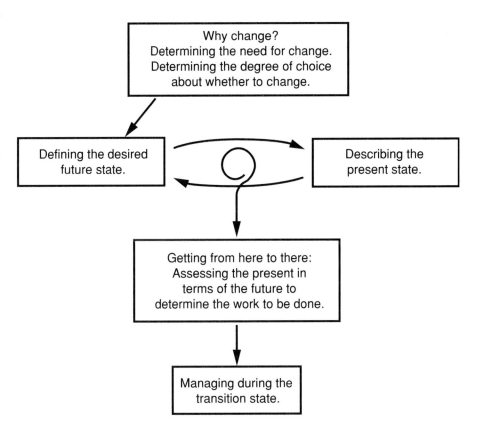

Fig. 6.1. Taken from Beckhard R and Harris R Organizational transitions (Fig. 4.1 page 31). © 1987, 1997. Addison Wesley Longman Inc. Reprinted by permission of Addison Wesley Longman.

All of these will influence the values that organisations adopt and will be similarly reflected in corporate objectives. Corporate objectives provide the general direction of an organisation's development. These are then translated into tasks that specify measurable goals and success criteria. It is clear that with the increasing responsibility of the Chief Executive for quality, the importance of effective clinical practice will be reflected in the organisation's objectives. Each service will need to identify the practical steps to be taken to deliver on this agenda successfully and support the change processes.

Change stakeholders

Within any service there are key players – some if not all will have an interest in the area of change (see Fig. 6.2). Therefore it is important to identify these individuals early to ensure they have an impact in shaping projects and thus own the process of change.

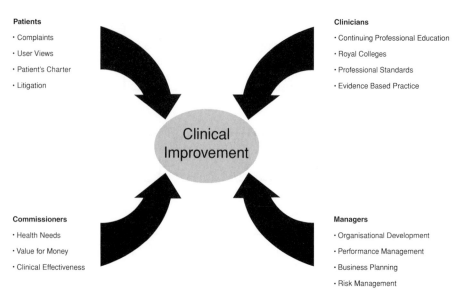

Patients
· Complaints
· User Views
· Patient's Charter
· Litigation

Clinicians
· Continuing Professional Education
· Royal Colleges
· Professional Standards
· Evidence Based Practice

Commissioners
· Health Needs
· Value for Money
· Clinical Effectiveness

Managers
· Organisational Development
· Performance Management
· Business Planning
· Risk Management

Fig. 6.2 Change stakeholders and influences.

Each stakeholder will have their own individual strategy and mission, and are likely to have hidden agendas. It is essential to secure support and commitment of all the stakeholders, as this will make change much easier. However, this is not easy, as there are always political issues that influence the degree of co-operation across functional barriers at all levels. This is especially true in health services where there are a number of different professions, different departments and services and possibly different values (e.g. managers versus clinicians). As well as internal stakeholders there are also external groups who have a major say in how services are delivered. Not least are patients and their advocates who are in effect the consumers of any change. Other external stakeholders include Health Authorities and Local Authorities, Professional Bodies, contractors, insurance agencies (i.e. CNST). While it may not be necessary to involve all of these directly in developing a change strategy, it is essential to elicit and consider each stakeholder's view.

Agreeing priorities

In the NHS there is a tendency to try and manage many different agendas and priorities which cannot all be progressed successfully. A method to systematically assess the potency for change of a goal and then apply a method of prioritisation is essential.

 This will help the service decide whether or not to even attempt to initiate change (i.e. few stakeholders support the goal).

▶ Secondly the service will be able to agree the relative priority of each goal and therefore how much energy and resource to give it.

There are various ways in which this could be done. One way to do this would be to develop a matrix grid with the degree of potency listed vertically and the change areas listed across the top.

Describing the future

Earlier in this chapter we described the need for Trusts to identify a set of objectives based on a vision of what the organisation wants to achieve. This describes the corporate future of the Trust. Having agreed which goals to deliver, the management team for each service needs to be able to describe how the service will look once the goals have been achieved. This should include structures and processes, as well as the standards at which these are to be achieved.

This is an essential step as it allows each individual service to make sense and *tailor* a previously generic goal. In so doing, a list of characteristics is developed that describes an effective service. While individual services may have the same goal, each one is likely to have a number of different characteristics, unique to their own setting.

An example of this would be if an Obstetric unit and an Anaesthetic service both identified the goal 'to ensure full implementation of Clinical Risk Management by xxxx'. Both services would have to describe the characteristics that achieved full implementation of clinical risk management. Both services are likely to have common characteristics that are corporately driven (i.e. a service policy, an incident reporting procedure, the consent process, etc.). However, the obstetric unit is likely to describe a policy on communication between midwives and medical staff, specific standards relating to *Changing Childbirth* (1993),[12] staffing levels on the labour ward, competencies in CTG interpretation, obstetric incident triggers. The anaesthetic service is likely to have policies on the maintenance and availability of anaesthetic equipment, a description of how the National Confidential Enquiry into Perioperative Death (NCEPOD)[13] reports are to be implemented, standards relating to pre-assessment and recovery, etc.

In collating a list of characteristics the service has to consider the two questions:

▶ What are the right things we should be doing?

▶ How well should we be doing them?

Identifying the right things to do

Trying to identify the right things to do is no easy task. Even today with national and international bodies commissioned to review and recommend good clinical practices there are still many grey areas where research studies are inconclusive.[14] The purpose of this chapter is not to list the various sources of clinical effectiveness information,[15] this is described in Chapter 14, or describe the process of validating research findings;

this has been done extensively elsewhere.[16] This section highlights the need to describe the future. The benefits of doing this are clear:

▶ *Overcomes resistance*: Having decided on characteristics that describe effective clinical services it is easy to see where individuals can fit themselves into future scenarios which they can then work with their colleagues to achieve.

▶ *Clarifies purpose*: By clarifying the purpose of the change it reduces uncertainty amongst clinical teams and allows them to begin to own the change.

▶ *Provides a focus for positive action*: By identifying corporate objectives and accompanying goals and values that support them, it allows all concerned to forward plan rather than dwell on short-termism and problem solving. It allows them to identify practical steps, formulate timescales and decide on priorities.

Setting standards

Having identified the right things to do it also is important to set standards that can be subsequently audited to give feedback on performance. By and large standards ensure ownership within the service or team. However, since the inception of clinical audit standards have notably been mainly used within the nursing profession[17] and then have often been misused focusing on short term attainment rather that continuous improvement.[18] For standards to be meaningful they must follow the SMART acronym:

S – Specific
M – Measurable
A – Achievable
R – Realistic
T – Timed

This means that all the service characteristics must be assigned an appropriate standard that specifies a measurable, which is realistic and achievable in terms of the capacity, capability and the culture of the service. The first obstetric unit goal could be incorporated with a standard as follows:

> The obstetric unit will have developed and implemented a policy with all clinical staff on communications between midwifery and medical staff during acute obstetric care by xx/yy/zz.

The effectiveness of implementing such a standard can then be measured using traditional clinical audit tools.

Assessing the current situation

Clinical teams must establish where they are now. How effective is their clinical practice? How much is evidence based? To determine this teams must draw on all

Table 6.1.

Area	Information Requirement	Information Source
Clinical Risk Management	• Trigger event reporting • Incident reports • Clinical Risk Assessment • Documentation Audit Results • Indicator information (mortality, complication rates)	Risk Management Database Annual Risk Assessment Routine monthly audits PAS analysis
Environmental Issues	• Incident statistics • Risk Assessments	Risk Management Database Annual Risk Assessment
Claims Management	• Claims data • Contingent liability by specialty	Risk Management Database
Professional Education	• CME/CPD Register • Colleges Curriculum	Clinical Directors log Colleges educational section
Consumer Expectations	• Complaints data, by consultant/ service/category • Suggestions • User surveys • Audit results	Risk Management Database Focus groups Local audit results
Employee Views	• Employee surveys • Leavers interviews • Briefing/open meetings • Staff side meetings	Routine survey results Sample interviews within service
Clinical Effectiveness	• NICE • Confidential enquiries • Clinical Indicators	Systematic reviews
Clinical Efficiency	• Readmission Rates • Patient's Charter results • Benchmarking data	CHKS and other benchmarking groups

available information. Assessing the future and the present state must work hand in hand. Standards can be clarified when existing performance is established, similarly a strategic goal in a particular area helps to identify information needs and provokes the question: '*is this a real issue for us?*'.

Using baseline information

Table 6.1 suggests a list of areas and information requirements that would need to be considered when identifying issues that require improved performance.

It is important that when we consider 'where we are now' we do not only look at crude indicators (e.g. Activity data, Incident reporting, Complaint information, etc.). Employee motivation, workload, stress and capability for change are all essential parts of the equation of making change happen.

Having identified both 'where we are now' and 'where we want to get to' it follows that we should easily be able to define what needs changing and what does not. The next step therefore is to develop an agenda for action, which specifies the key steps in 'getting from here to there'.

How to make change happen

Many excellent texts have been written describing how to effect change using a project management framework. This section does not replicate these, but rather attempts to describe how this approach can be applied to the implementation of clinical governance and clinical audit, highlighting key success factors.

If the management team is to be successful it first needs to translate the goals and characteristics into a meaningful project. To deliver the project will require both teamwork and effective leadership. A project team should be selected on the basis of skills, experience and an ability to carry out the work involved.

Any multidisciplinary team should begin by asking themselves the following questions:

▶ What do we need to do?

▶ How are we going to do it?

▶ When do we need to do each part?

▶ Where are we going to do it?

▶ What are we **not** going to do?

▶ How will we know how well we have done it?

Having begun to answer some of these questions the team should be able to derive detailed plans and schedules to carry out the work. Individual responsibilities are decided and agreed. The work plans that are designed should identify solutions to bring about change, the mechanism by which this solution is to be implemented and success criteria to show implementation has been successful.

Example

One of the goals of a surgical unit is to further develop clinical risk management. The service decides that one of the effective characteristics of this would be good clinical record keeping and therefore sets some standards of performance for all clinical staff. It is known that record keeping in the unit is not good, and this has been clearly demonstrated in a number of clinical negligence claims that could not be defended because of poor documentation.

The unit set up a project team to change record keeping practice. The team consisted of a consultant surgeon (project lead), service manager, junior doctor (research registrar), ward manager, staff nurse and a clinical improvement facilitator.

The above example describes a balanced multidisciplinary project team with the relevant knowledge, skills and abilities to deliver the project goal. The project team should be a mixture of people at different levels that represent what happens in reality within the clinical setting. By and large it is junior medical and nursing staff who see and care for the majority of patients most of the time and as such they are the ones who are the main record keepers. It is therefore essential that they should be represented in any project team for two reasons.

 They can bring a realistic view to the team on why things are not done right and the barriers to effective record keeping.

 Secondly they can advise on tactics to overcome barriers and act as educators or use peer pressure with other medical and nursing staff to help implement the new standards.

The project team is therefore about doing the job of changing practice; it is not about trying to accommodate stakeholders' views and expectations. To help confirm this, it is useful to establish basic ground rules with the project team to which they all agree and literally sign. These might include attendance at meetings, administrating the project, communications and dissemination of information. This type of approach has been successfully employed within our own Trust.

Identifying and implementing solutions

During the last decade a number of quality solutions have been identified all of which have their champions and critics. Most notable of these are Integrated Care Management[19] and Clinical Guidelines.[20] Both of these initiatives are described in more depth within other chapters.

All or some aspects of these tools can be utilised within a project plan. In the above example the unit may decide to re-engineer the way in which their records are handled so that fewer people handle the records which makes them easier to locate and retrieve. Similarly, the unit may decide to introduce a number of care pathways which replace the existing documentation with standardised multidisciplinary care plans for particular surgical conditions such as breast cancer, varicose veins, etc. Lastly the unit may agree to publish all future clinical guidelines with a section on record keeping and the need to document particular aspects of care within high-risk conditions.

Whatever solution is selected the action plans must describe the process of implementation, i.e.

 What are the policies, procedures and/or guidelines that are to be used to support this change?

 How are they to be launched and disseminated?

 What educational initiatives are to be used to raise awareness and ensure understanding?

Monitoring performance

The other question that the project team will need to consider is *'what measures will be used to evaluate how effective they have been in achieving the goal'*. This is the area, which has traditionally been associated with the measurement phase in clinical audit. If SMART standards have been set at the outset of each project then monitoring these should be relatively straightforward. It is essential, however, that the team's project plan identifies the key steps in this process, i.e.

▶ Data to be collected that test standards.

▶ Method of data collection; prospective, retrospective.

▶ Design of proformas.

▶ Who will collect data, from where and how much?

▶ Who will analyse data, using what methods?

▶ How will results be reported and performance subsequently monitored?

Having measured performance, the project team needs to feed back the results to the management team and other stakeholders via a previously agreed process. This may be an annual review of directorate objectives or part of a routine performance monitoring mechanism. The management team would have to consider the results in the light of new areas of work the service has been asked to do or that have arisen out of performance monitoring. They would have to decide if the performance of the service was acceptable in reaching the required standards. If it is, then should higher standards be set and the change cycle repeated? If the service has failed to reach standards the management team must consider why this may have happened. Questions they may wish to ask include:

▶ Was a correct assessment made of the nature of change?

▶ Was commitment established and resistance overcome?

▶ Were standards realistic and achievable?

▶ Was the change process well planned, was it explicit and detailed and was it effectively communicated?

▶ Are the performance results valid?

Clinical governance and audit: Making it happen

The process described above highlights the practical approach to using clinical audit within a change management model. In order to make this happen, a Trust will need to have a strategy that brings together all the systems for quality improvement under the umbrella of clinical governance. Some of the key questions that form the basis of this strategy are:

▶ What structures and processes are needed to support a strategy for continuous quality improvements?

▶ What are the competencies that are required by all levels of staff to deliver continuous quality improvements?

▶ What needs to happen at an operational level for quality improvements to happen?

▶ What are the information sources for assessing service quality and deciding priorities for action?

▶ What monitoring arrangements are needed to ensure change occurs?

Organising for clinical audit

Traditionally many organisations have organised clinical audit activity around a central Clinical Audit Committee. The Committee's role varies from Trust to Trust, however, they often have responsibilities for co-ordinating, monitoring, and advising on corporate audit activity. In the advent of clinical governance the role and function of such committees are likely to change.

As Trusts become accountable for the continuous improvement of their services, systems will evolve which will manage this process. It quite naturally follows that the Clinical Audit Committee in many organisations could develop into the local clinical governance group. The earlier part of this chapter described how clinical audit could be used as a mechanism for setting standards, changing practice and monitoring performance. If this is the case, then a Trust's Audit Committee should be a key player in all of these roles and will have to be multidisciplinary. It should be made up not only of doctors, nurses and therapists, but also senior managers and directors of the organisation who work in partnership with clinicians, to improve and change practice. The committee will also require representation from colleagues in the local Health Authority, local GPs and also a user or patient representative. If the committee is to be accountable for the quality of clinical practice, it must also have the power to influence and change practice. This would represent a significant change in the role of the committee, which for many organisations has been purely advisory up until recently.

Whilst the Clinical Audit Committee is highly important, little will change in practice without local services working hand in hand with the committee to improve performance. Services need to set up their local arrangements, which are governed by the Clinical Audit Committee. A Corporate framework for Clinical Audit and change management needs to be agreed, and this needs to be implemented within each service. The service then needs to self-assess on a routine basis, how well it is implementing the framework, along with other policies and procedures to enable improvement in practice. In this way the Clinical Audit Committee can accredit each services performance, not on how well it changes practice, but on how well it has implemented systems that enable change.

Developing competencies

The agenda for change that has been created by clinical governance is enormous, and will require effective leadership, team working at all levels of the organisation, and above all multi-professional education and training.

Clinical Audit has now been used within Health services for a number of years, and yet there is still confusion about what exactly clinical audit means. For some audit is about measuring performance, for others it is about achieving quality standards and some clinicians still see audit as part of a research agenda. To begin to overcome such diversity will require organisations to devise and run multidisciplinary training programmes on clinical audit. The programme should include modules on the concept of audit, identifying and prioritising activities, setting standards and establishing criteria, writing action plans and enabling change. With the advent of national service frameworks, and the likelihood of national audit projects, it is likely that services will be required to practically undertake audits, much more than they have been required to previously. The responsibility for undertaking projects and enabling change, will be explicitly part of service delivery, with clinical audit departments enabling and enhancing the services potential.

It is important that training is delivered to all levels of the organisation and not just frontline staff. Trust Board members and Senior Directors must also understand and sign-up to audit so that they can facilitate change and prioritise resources accordingly.

Teamworking

Earlier in this book leadership was described as being essential in changing practice, however, one of the characteristics of any effective leader is to align their team to a common goal. Any patient who comes into hospital is likely to have contact with administrative staff, nurses, doctors and possibly therapists, as well as a whole host of other technical staff. All these staff are vital cogs in the machine that produces effective outcomes, yet all may have different aims. A doctor may be concerned with getting a person medically stable so that they can return home as soon as possible; a therapist may be wondering whether the patient will be able to function safely at home; while a nurse may be trying to provide the best possible care to enable their recovery. In order to change practice all of these differing aims need to be realigned to one common goal. To do this the team must have a mutual understanding of each other's role and how this contributes to achieving the goal. Each profession within a clinical team will need to recognise their interdependence on each other and be willing to work together to achieve common standards. Teams that work effectively require honesty, respect of each other and equity. Most readers will by now recognise that this is no easy task given the cultural history of the Health service and its different professional groups.

For some time clinical audit has been led by clinicians, often medical staff. All too often local audit leads have been chosen for their enthusiasm and interest rather than their leadership ability.[21] Managers have not been encouraged or actively participated in clinical audit. This is partly due to a lack of knowledge and understanding,[22] but also because clinicians perceived their involvement as a threat.[23] The result of this is that all too often audit has been seen as a peripheral activity rather than a fundamental part of professional development. Bowden (1996)[24] suggests that for clinical audit to be effective it must have the support and active involvement of managers for the following reasons:

▶ Managers have a responsibility to provide a suitable environment and an obligation to develop a process through which audit can take place.

▶ Managers create the culture for change within an organisation.

▶ They often control the resources through which change can take place.

It is likely that senior clinicians will lead the governance agenda, while managers will be responsible for making the processes work and for producing results. It is naïve to suggest that existing clinical directors are qualified to produce change or that managers have the skills to manage teams that change clinical practice. These and other skills will have to be learned by both clinicians and managers. Both will need to understand each other's roles, their motivation, and work in unison if they are to be effective in improving quality of care for their patients.

Historically dedicated time has been set aside within Trusts for clinical audit activity. At best this has been used for planning which audit projects should be undertaken within a particular service. In other areas medical staff have used this time to describe the results of audit projects they may have undertaken.[26] Multidisciplinary teams have spent very little of this time considering where their services need to improve in line with their service goals, and what common learning and education needs the team may have. However, such an approach could harness ownership amongst the team and create an agenda for action. Clinical Improvement Groups that can take on this role have been described in Chapter 3.

Information Management

Information has two key purposes. It assists in the decision making process and secondly it helps to monitor the progress of decisions that have been made. Information is therefore fundamental to making change happen.

Information systems within Trusts have tended to evolve out of corporate information need, and as such have been business and finance led. Clinical information systems have been given much less priority within the 'contract culture' and have often been developed on a piecemeal basis around specific service need (i.e. diagnostics services). It is therefore not uncommon to find Trusts with a plethora of systems having often been developed in isolation, with little integration.

Clinical governance will create a tremendous drive for information on clinical performance. This will require an integrated solution whereby all the clinical team can easily provide clinical data that can then be quickly transformed into meaningful information. This has been done on a small scale in such things as incident reporting and complaint management, however, initiatives such as National Service Frameworks and the National Performance Framework are likely to drive IM&T strategy at a pace. To make this work will undoubtedly require the funding of new technologies as well as a huge investment in education and training. Solutions will have to be found to the age old problems of data collection and data management. Technologies such as smart cards,[25] clinical workstations[26] and electronic patient records[27] have been tried and tested but have had little impact to date.

Systems will also have to be developed that are designed to assure the Trust Board that clinical governance and audit arrangements are working and in place. Recommendations that arise out of audit projects will all require explicit leads and dates which will then need to be actioned. Each service will need to monitor the progress of the action plans reporting variance to the clinical governance group and Trust Board. It is envisaged that similar systems will have to be developed for risk management, complaints and claims management and workforce planning. Information issues are discussed in detail in Chapter 13.

The future of support services: change agents

During the early 1990s we have seen the rise in quality assurance departments and resource management units. Complaints departments and customer affairs units then joined these services. It was and still is not uncommon for these initiatives to be managed centrally but often separately by the Trust's Director of Nursing. With the advent of medical and latterly clinical audit, audit departments began to develop sometimes subsuming existing quality improvement services or more commonly running alongside them. These were again sometimes managed by the Director of Nursing, but were often led by the Trust's Medical Director who also chaired the Clinical Audit Committee. Most recently we have seen the rise in clinical risk management and clinical effectiveness units.

In many Trusts all these functions have worked co-operatively together, although often on separate initiatives. Operational services have also been confused as to how this jigsaw fits together, setting up clinical audit meetings separate from quality development forums and clinical risk management groups. What has hindered further development in this area is the lack of a corporate wide strategy on quality improvement, which would identify the key roles each initiative has to play and the interfaces between them such as a clinical governance framework. Once the future state has been identified, it is likely that new roles will naturally emerge for central support functions.

For many Trusts the clinical audit department's role has been to provide project management, and technical advice on the measurement phase of the audit cycle, with the department administrating and reporting on all projects undertaken. Some departments have extended their role to include clinical effectiveness and are proactively involved in the setting of standards with the whole team. In order for clinical governance to work and for change to happen, departments like clinical audit will also need to change, with different competencies and skills required from their staff.

Overview of quality improvement initiatives

There will be a need for clinical departments to have an overview of all the quality improvement initiatives from clinical risk management, complaints and health & safety to clinical effectiveness. There will be a need for specialists in these areas to act as internal consultants and provide corporate wide advice. These specialists will need to work together as a team, regardless of whether they are managed by the same person. This will require much greater matrix working within the organisation and a sharing of resources between corporate functions. It is also likely that there will be a need for people to have specialist change management skills and have a broad understanding of each of the quality initiatives so that they can facilitate projects and enable services to change. Clinical Improvement Facilitators will be employed to work with services and help them through the process rather than work for a service. This will mean that less technical skills will be required and competencies such as negotiation, training, planning and conflict management will become increasingly in demand. Such facilitators would play a key role in Clinical Improvement Groups acting as an expert to the group on quality improvement. This role could be seen in the same light as that of a finance or a human resources manager acting as a professional adviser in their respective fields, but with the operational service managing the budgets and developing the staff. The role of the facilitator may also include a governance function to ensure that operational services are actively implementing the right policies and following the right processes set out within the Trust's clinical governance framework.

References

1   Department of Health. *A First Class Service*. HMSO. 1998.
2   Department of Health. Medical Audit – Working Paper No 6. *Working for Patients*. HMSO. 1989.
3   Royal College of Physicians. Medical Audit. A First Report. *What, Why, and How*. Royal College of Physicians, London. 1989.
4   NHSE. Clinical Audit 1994/95 and beyond, EL(94)20. HMSO. 1994.
5   Berger A. (1998). *Why doesn't audit work?* British Medical Journal; 316: 875–876.
6   Shaw C. (1989). *Medical Audit: A Hospital Handbook*. Kings Fund Centre, KFC 89/11, London.
7   Walshe K and Coles Y. (1993). *Medical Audit in need of evaluation*. Quality in Health Care 2: 189–190.
8   Malby B. (1995). Getting started on Audit. In *Clinical Audit for Nurses and Therapists*. Scutari Press, London.
9   Rogers B. (1983). *Diffusion of innovation*, 3rd ed. Free Press, New York.
10 Broome A. (1990). *Managing Change*. Macmillan, London.
11 Beckhard R and Harris R. (1987). *Organizational Transitions*, 2nd ed. Addison-Wesley, Reading, Massachusetts.
12 Department of Health. *Changing Childbirth*. Report of the Expert Maternity Group. HMSO. 1993.
13 Gallimore SC, Hoile RW, Ingram GS and Sherry KM. (1997). The Report of the National Confidential Enquiry into Perioperative Deaths. NCEPOD, London.
14 Naylor CD. (1995). Grey zones of clinical practice: some limits to evidence-based medicine. *Lancet*, 345: 840–842.
15 NHSE. *Promoting Clinical Effectiveness*. A framework for action, HMSO. 1996.
16 Miles A, Lugon M and Polychronis A. (1996). *The Development of Quality in Clinical Practice II: The Derivation and Implementation of Clinical Standards, Guidelines and Research Evidence*. In Miles A and Lugon M. (1996). *Effective Clinical Practice*. Blackwell Science, Oxford.
17 Kemp N and Richardson E. (1993). *Quality Assurance in Nursing Practice*. Butterworth-Heinemann Ltd, Oxford.
18 Malby B. (1995). Linking Resource Management Quality and Audit. In *Clinical Audit for Nurses and Therapists*. Scutari Press, London.
19 Wilson JH. (1996). *Integrated Care Management: The Path to Success*. Butterworth-Heinemann, Oxford.
20 Grimshaw J, Fremantle N, Wallace S, Russell L, Hurwitz B. Watt I, Long A and Sheldon T. (1995). *Developing and implementing Clinical Practice Guidelines*. Quality in Health Care 4: 55–64.
21 Scally G and Donaldson LJ. (1998). *Clinical Governance and the drive for quality improvement in the new NHS in England*. British Medical Journal, 317: 61–65.
22 Coe P. (1994). Management's legitimate interests in clinical audit. In Hopkins A. (1996). *Professional and Managerial Aspects of Clinical Audit*. The Royal College of Physicians, London.
23 McIntyre N. (1995). *Evaluation in Clinical Practice – problems, principles and precedents*. Journal of Evaluation in Clinical Practice 1: 5–13.

24   Bowden D. (1996). Partnerships in Clinical Audit: Senior Management and the Clinical Professions. In Miles A and Lugon M. (1996). *Effective Clinical Practice*. Blackwell Science, Oxford.

25   Cross M. (1998). *Putting Health on the Cards*. Health Service Journal. 5 February: 24–25.

26   Jones A. (1997). *The Benefits of the Integrated Clinical Workstation Programme*. Winchester & Eastleigh Healthcare NHS Trust.

27   Paul R. (1997). Electronic Patient Record Project. Burton Hospitals NHS Trust.

▶7

Clinical Risk Management

Jonathan Secker-Walker

The consultation document 'A first class service',[1] subsequent to the government's White Paper *The New NHS. Modern. Dependable*[2] places clinical risk reduction programmes and critical incident reporting as some of the main components of clinical governance.

Risk management is an accepted function within industrial and financial institutions. Clear evidence that clinical risk management reduces the number of accidents to patients is hard to come by although common sense would suggest that early identification of accidents and speedy settlement of claims or complaints save money and are inherently better for patients. Hospitals in Maryland that had implemented programmes regarding physician and nurse responsibilities in quality assurance and risk management have been shown by Morlock[3] to reduce both the number of claims and the quantum awarded. Risks associated with safety to staff are believed to be reduced by adherence to Health and Safety regulations whilst meeting standards proposed by the Central Negligence Scheme for Trusts, the Welsh Risk Pool or other insurer is likely to improve patient safety and has the advantage of reducing premiums.

Management of clinical risk tends to be associated with the cost of clinical negligence which, for the NHS, is currently around £200 million annually. Whilst this is currently less than the budget of one of the larger teaching hospitals, the rate of increase in litigation and the value of awards appears inexorable. Several studies suggest that whilst the rate of negligent accidents appears to affect around 1% of in-patients, the overall rate of injuries or adverse outcomes as a result of medical or clinical management is considerably greater. It has been estimated at about 4–5% of in-patients in two USA studies,[4,5] 16.6% in a recent Australian study[6] and as high as 45% in two acute surgical units in Chicago and Florida, of which 17.7% were considered serious. Analysis of these surgical events suggests that nearly 40% were due to poor individual technical performance or judgement, 15% due to failure of communication and 10% due to inappropriate administrative decisions.[7] To extrapolate the findings of Leape and Brennan et al[8] who defined an adverse event as 'an unintended injury that was caused by medical management and that resulted in measurable disability' to an average NHS Trust treating 50,000 in-patients would suggest that in any one year there would be 1850 adverse events, 48 patients permanently disabled and 251 deaths, of which about half would be due to negligence (0.25% of all in-patients). Thus, whilst the cost of clinical negligence is a significant and growing problem, the overall cost of patient and staff injuries to the NHS in terms of increased days in hospital, extra investigations or days on sick leave for staff, probably accounts for a significant percentage of the overall NHS budget.

Accident investigation

Accidents have been more thoroughly investigated in industry and transport than in clinical practice, although the work of Cooper,[9] Gaba,[10] Runciman,[11] in anaesthesia is extremely important. It is a reasonable assumption that the vast majority of staff working in healthcare are committed to providing a service of high quality and yet human error of one sort or another appears to be responsible for about 70% of accidents, equipment failure accounting for perhaps 15–20%, whilst poor design of equipment, lack of policies for uniform equipment or inadequate training in its use is often implicated.

Most clinicians who have been involved in an accident involving a patient will recognise that it was seldom a single isolated event but a constellation of numerous factors, many outside the clinician's control, that ultimately led to the error. Reason[12] quotes Mr Justice Sheen's report[13] into the capsizing of the *Herald of Free Enterprise* in 1987 which highlights the distinction between *active human failures* – the sailor who did not shut the bow doors – and *latent human failures* – the inadequate organisational policies or inappropriate decisions that sculpted the environment in which active failures were more likely to thrive. These *latent human failures* can be likened to resident pathogens just biding their time for appropriate conditions in which to strike. Organisations such as hospitals recognise that human beings are prone to error, making mistakes and breaking or violating rules or protocols, and put in place *defences* – monitoring equipment or procedures – that reduce the likelihood of human fallibility leading to an accident.

The risks of intravenous infusion devices will be familiar to most doctors and nurses and usually account for a significant proportion of adverse medication incidents. This is a good example of medical practice moving more rapidly than the organisation's ability to respond to change and introduce appropriate defences. Not only is there often no uniformity of equipment on the wards – let alone the hospital – but permanent staff often receive no formal training in the use of the different syringe pumps and temporary staff practically never. A further problem inherent in these methods of drug administration is that the solutions are more concentrated and therefore mathematical error – a decimal point perhaps – may have serious consequences. Some clinical staff find maths difficult and drug companies provide drug concentrations in different formats; mg/ml, per cent solutions, 1 in 1000, etc.

The trajectory of an accident can be illustrated in Reason's model[12] which neatly demonstrates the main components that may be partly responsible. (Fig. 7.1).

Risk management and human factors

Clinical risk management is a framework designed to help identify the varied causes of latent failure, inadequate or inappropriate defences and active human failure. Making the link between risk management and human factors research into industrial, transport or medical accidents, would appear to persuade sceptical doctors to support concepts and methods of managing risk. For many years aviation has learnt detailed lessons from its disasters and near-misses to make flying safer; medicine can use risk management to achieve the same end.

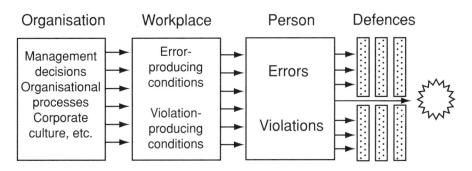

Fig. 7.1 Modelling organisational accidents. Reproduced with permission from James Reason. © BMJ Publishing.

The definition of an adverse incident, however, needs to be broader than that used by Leape and Brennan[8] in order to collect information related to likely precursors of accidents, environmental conditions (lack of staff, communication failures) and evidence of failed defences (inadequate pre-operative assessment, no oximeters available in endoscopy) as well as actual accidents to patients. Such a definition may be as broad as:

> any occurrence which is not consistent with the routine care of the patient or the
> routine operation of the institution, whilst a near-miss can be defined as an
> occurrence which but for luck or skilful management would in all probability have
> become an incident.

Clinical risk management, with these human factor concepts as its foundation, aims to achieve four principal objectives.

1. Identification of organisational, system failures or defence inadequacies so that managers can act to remedy the situation before an accident occurs. Incident data may indicate areas where accidents to patients are likely to happen if no management action is taken – for example an ICU with unclear responsibilities between surgeons, physicians and anaesthetists. This proactive management of risk should aim to continuously monitor the capacity for latent failure within the organisation.
2. The collection of records as soon after an accident as possible. Prompt incident reporting allows risk managers to collect relevant records, pathology forms, x-rays, CTGs and witness statements relating to incidents considered liable to lead to a claim – for example a low apgar baby. This is in contrast to the common problem of trying to seek evidence several years after the event, with the result that some defensible claims cannot be defended for lack of contemporary records.
3. By providing early warning of possible claims, incident reporting allows up-to-date evidence to be used by the Trust to consider whether to settle or fight a possible claim or resolve a clinical complaint – many of which may be the precursor to a claim. Honesty with patients and a move to an early equitable

settlement (where appropriate) is usually better for the patient and staff involved and less costly in legal fees for the hospital.

4. Finally, early incident reporting allows a structured, objective examination of the facts surrounding a serious event relating to both active and latent human failures or mechanical breakdown or combinations of all three. This enables the hospital to learn lessons so that safety can be enhanced and future practice improved.

Staff working at the hospital coal-face are a valuable and informed source of knowledge about risk in their area and the collection of information about such perceived risks through an incident reporting system provides essential data for managers. The willingness to report near-misses and actual accidents soon after the event are also essential ingredients of the risk management process.

It is a fundamental tenet of the risk management that, whilst overall responsibility for risk management lies with the Chief Executive of the Trust, the general managers, clinical directors, business and directorate managers must accept that the management of risks in their wards and departments is one of their key responsibilities and should be explicit in their agreed objectives.

Disciplinary action

Threat of discipline for staff does not encourage the early reporting of incidents. This means that the benefits of investigation and learning from the event tend not to be realised. Many hospitals treat groups of clinical staff differently in terms of discipline after an accident. After an error, junior medical staff may be admonished by their consultant whilst nursing staff may face disciplinary action. It is not uncommon for these two approaches to be applied to the same incident. If a member of staff risks disciplinary action, a report on their personnel file or the loss of their job, they are less likely to feel like owning up to a mistake. Equity demands that all professional disciplines are treated in a similar fashion. The hospital or healthcare organisation needs to empower all staff to report incidents without the fear of disciplinary action and this decision is an essential first step in any risk management programme. The Chief Executive should make it clear that no disciplinary action will result from reporting incidents, mistakes or near-misses, with the proviso that an agreement will be reached with management regarding the specific problems which will be the exception to the general rule of non-disciplinary action. Such issues which would continue to lead to disciplinary action would include criminal or malicious activities (including malicious reporting), acts of gross misconduct and repeated errors or violations.

The Medical Director

It is usually a prerequisite for the success of clinical risk management that the Medical Director of the institution is committed to the process and acts as chairman of the Risk Management and Incident and Claims Review Committees. Before the advent of clinical governance, this may not have always been the case, but would now appear inevitable. A combination of a Medical Director and Director of Nursing Service working in harmony is a potent recipe for success.

The Risk Manager

The Risk Manager should help design, implement and coordinate the Trust's Clinical Risk Management Programme, involving risk detection, assessment, prevention and appraisal.

The responsibilities of the Trust's Clinical Risk Manager should include the promotion of relationships within the hospital to develop understanding of and support for risk management activities, including implemention of hospital-wide risk education and prevention programmes as well as hospital-wide induction programmes in risk management for all new employees. In addition an important task is to work with clinical staff and managers to ensure the Trust meets the Standards for Risk Management laid down in due course by relevant Insurers, which is likely to include organisation-wide clinical risk assessments, similar to the process carried out for health and safety risk. The Risk Manager cannot be expected to achieve compliance with all the standards alone but should be seen to be responsible for coordinating the effort.

The development and maintenance of the adverse incident reporting system with agreement from the Risk Management Committee as to reporting policy, the nature and frequency of reports is another important part of the job. The Risk Manager should review each day's incident forms before they are given to the data entry secretary. This allows significant incidents to be immediately followed up or brought to the attention of the relevant manager. Any serious incident should be reported to the Medical Director immediately. Regular feedback by the Risk Manager of action taken as a result of incident reports to the staff who reported them is essential to maintain momentum.

Adverse incident evaluation

The Risk Manager is best placed to act as secretary to the Risk Management Committee and the Incident and Claims Review Committee and in this role can effectively coordinate the interlinking activities of these groups. As such the Risk Manager should work closely with the Complaints and Litigation Officers to ensure that the Trust coordinates its claims management as required by the Insurers and that the relevant data is regularly available to them. He or she should evaluate all adverse incidents that might lead to a claim and ensure the collection and safe storage of all relevant medical/nursing records, x-rays, images, pathology reports, tissue sections and witness statements, together with the addresses and telephone numbers of all relevant staff, including locums.

As secretary to the Incident and Claims Review Committee, the Risk Manager should ensure that regular reports required by the committee are available in due time, be responsible for the minutes and prepare the agenda in consultation with the Medical Director and liaise with the Complaints and Litigation Officers to provide appropriate papers to the Clinical Incident and Claims Review Committee. Finally the Risk Manager should establish close working relationships with health and safety staff and those working in clinical audit since many risk management issues cross the boundaries of these activities.

Incident reporting

It is not possible to identify accurately the full extent of the Trust's risk issues, without the full notification, recording, analysis and feedback of information, in relation to adverse incidents. There is an analogy likening hospital function to multiple slices of Swiss cheese (Reason 1996, personal communication) in constant brownian movement. Holes are randomly distributed throughout the cheese, representing latent failures and active failures. An adverse incident can be considered as the identification of a hole in the cheese which can then be blocked up, making an accident trajectory less likely (Fig. 7.2). Constant monitoring of incidents depends on staff reporting organisational process failures as well as their own errors and thus every effort must be made to avoid cover-ups of adverse incidents, mistakes or near misses. The overall approach within the Trust should be one of help and support to each other, rather than recrimination and blame. Every adverse incident which is reported should be seen as a chance to learn in order to improve the quality of care in the future.

The procedures and systems in place for the reporting and collection of untoward incidents and accidents must be simple, straightforward and understood by all staff. The use of a single incident form for all types of adverse event, both clinical, staff and non-clinical, is to be preferred. Simplicity of form design and clarity of destination promote compliance.

Healthcare organisations are usually organised in vertical formations (i.e. directorates), whilst many risk factors run horizontally across institutions. Individual departmental managers require a copy of the incident form for their own use, but another copy of all forms should be directed through one central point for analysis, not only vertically but horizontally, with that information then being disseminated to directorate level for action. This horizontal analysis is a central function of the Risk Management Committee and clinical data dissemination should

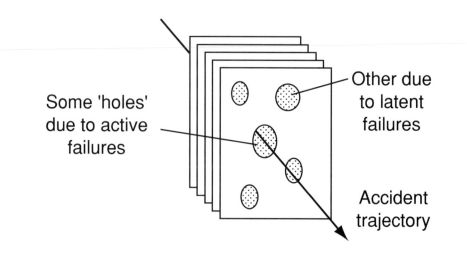

Some 'holes' due to active failures

Other due to latent failures

Accident trajectory

Fig. 7.2 Breached defences. Reproduced with permission from James Reason.

be conducted by the Risk Manager, who should liaise with directorates and monitor progress. Health & Safety staff and clinical risk management should adopt policies that ensure that each incident form is reviewed and directed to the appropriate destination for action.

IT requirements

Once the risk management programme is running, the risk management office may receive about 5–15 incident forms a day, although this is very variable. A large proportion of these will be slips and falls and other relatively minor incidents and discretion and experience is required of the Risk Manager in filtering out the significant from the insignificant. It is necessary to arrange an explicit flow path for the Incident Forms to ensure that incidents are all reviewed and graded by the Clinical Risk Manager before entry onto a database and that the appropriate forms are then received in a timely fashion by Health and Safety, Occupational Health and other departments. A suitable relational database is essential for the analysis of trends of incidents by directorate or department and for submitting reports to the Insurer. At the same time complaints and claims, both clinical and non-clinical, are best managed using appropriate software. An interactive system with incident, complaint and claims data together is of great use.

Indicators

A major component of the management of clinical risk is an agreed system for the reporting of clinically related patient incidents and near misses. Many core sets of Indicators have been developed, for example by the JCAHO[14] and the Maryland Hospital Association[15] in the USA and the medico-legal claims administrators LADD in South Australia.[16] MMI Companies Inc. after extensive research into its claims, have developed specialty specific indicators in perinatal care,[17] anaesthesia, surgery, emergency medicine and other specialties. The company has demonstrated a reduction in the number and value of claims if its simple guidelines are followed. Examples of its guidelines are a requirement to use fetal monitoring whenever oxytocin is used or to use oximetry whenever intravenous sedation is used.

One of the duties of the Risk Management Committee should be to review a list of 'indicators'. Most are self evidently the possible precursors of claims and whilst the core sets may apply to most specialties, individual specialties such as theatres and anaesthesia or paediatrics will wish to develop their own. (Examples in the Appendix) These, after consideration by the Committee, should be submitted to the clinical directors who will wish to discuss them with colleagues and modify them with their own particular specialty-specific indicators. It is important to recognise that the cause of many of these Indicators will be as a result of the patient's inherent pathology, but may also be precursors of claims or complaints. Once agreed by the clinical team they should be reported to the Risk Manager verbally, by fax or by using the Incident Report Form. It is of importance that the whole clinical team agrees the indicators for the department. Doctors and form filling are not natural partners and other clinical staff may have greater compliance; thus prior agreement as to what constitutes an incident or indicator should avoid one profession feeling reported on by another.

Once an indicator is reported, a judgement needs to be made about the significance of the incident. Serious events will require that the Serious Clinical Incident Procedure is instigated which should be a policy that is clearly described with the responsibilities and roles for the Medical Director, Director of Nursing and the Risk Manager and usually includes a formal inquiry. Other incidents are best served by a risk management meeting involving those concerned to establish the facts and make recommendations for the future. Sometimes recurring indicator data of a more minor nature will provide pointers to suggest that practice might perhaps be improved – for instance where a particular surgeon appears to have to admit more than the usual percentage of day-case surgery patients.

Data analysis and feedback

It is important that once there is sufficient quantity, the analysis of clinical data collected is reviewed centrally through the Central Risk Management Committee. This enables a proper focus to be given to the data received, in order to provide meaningful and useful information of trends and patterns of incidents occurring.

Most healthcare staff believe that hospital forms disappear into some sort of management black hole. The reporting of incidents/accidents increases if those sending in the reports are provided with some feedback on the action taken (or not) on the incidents concerned. Such *positive reinforcement* is essential for effective risk management and should be provided to the staff involved by the Risk Manager or their managers.

Risk Management Committee

The role of the Risk Management Committee, chaired by the Medical Director, should be to provide a systematic and strategic approach to the management of all clinical risks within the Trust. A significant role, once the Board has agreed a 'no-blame' culture is to ensure that staff reporting incidents or near-misses are not subject to discipline unless the behaviour is criminal, is malicious, constitutes gross misconduct or deviates from the Board's published policy. Other important functions are to decide the nature and form of regular reports derived from the incident database so that the committee can advise the Executive Officers and Trust Board on urgent risk management issues and make recommendations as to solutions. Education and training in risk management, which should be a continuing process for all staff (and especially at induction) needs to be overseen by the committee which should also ensure that a library of appropriate literature is available and that Medical Device warnings or pertinent pharmaceutical advice reaches relevant personnel.

The committee should establish and maintain a timetable for an ongoing programme of risk assessment throughout the Trust and receive reports from areas that have been surveyed.

Other tasks falling to the committee should be to monitor the level of compliance with the Insurer's risk management standards, to receive regular relevant reports from the Control of Infection Committee, the Clinical Audit Committee, the Drug & Therapeutics Committee, the Resuscitation Committee, the Blood Transfusion Committee and other monitors of clinical performance.

Claims management

Most Trusts have an excess level with their insurer, below which they have to pay costs and quantum. The issue for most Trusts is whether to continue *handling* claims for their solicitors to *manage*, or whether the Trust should start to actively *manage* its claims where it is felt to be appropriate.

The positive management of clinical incidents, complaints and actual civil legal actions brought against a Trust is an integral part of the risk management process. Management of such events serves four purposes:

1. It saves considerable sums of money by assembling material evidence and witness statements as close in time to the incident as possible.
2. It can obtain swift resolution of complaints or early settlement with plaintiffs where clinical care is considered to be below standard, preferably before both sides' lawyers get involved.
3. Where necessary, by getting early expert opinion, it empowers lawyers acting for the Trust to fight unwarranted claims forcefully, thereby reducing the frequency of going to court.
4. It reduces the trauma to patients and staff of the litigation process.

The organisation needs to develop a mechanism to take an early view of the standard of care delivered after a patient accident, claim or complaint and then make a decision about a satisfactory resolution of the problem. Because swift resolution of appropriate cases depends on early warning from incident reporting by staff that an error has occurred, it is very important that the Risk Manager and the Complaints and Litigation Officers work closely together – preferably from offices in close proximity.

Incident & Claims Review Committee (see also Chapter 10)

Formation of an Incident & Claims Review Committee (ICRC) provides a mechanism for taking an early view of the degree to which the complainant or plaintiff is correct or incorrect in the assertion that care was below the standard expected. Experience suggests that about a quarter of incidents are definitely defensible, a quarter indefensible and half are less easy to determine. For the areas of uncertainty, the ICRC, may choose to agree a list of external specialists, recognised as leaders in their field, who are prepared to provide expert opinion to the committee to assist in its deliberations. Outside expert opinion can also be useful in areas where the ICRC feels that the standard of care was appropriate and that the claim should be resolutely defended.

The Incident & Claims Review Committee is created to assess the quality of care provided to patients in the Trust and to recommend to the Clinical Directors changes and modifications in the rendering of care that reduces risk and leads to improved practice in the future. A secondary responsibility is to assist the Medical Director, the Chief Executive and the Trust's lawyers in determining whether the care provided met, fell below or exceeded the established standard of care.

The Committee's role is to:

1. Review relevant cases where disclosure of notes has been sought by a plaintiff.
2. Review clinical incidents where Risk Management considers litigation possible.
3. Monitor the progress of litigation already underway.
4. Recommend improvements in practice arising from consideration of the cases.

In the light of the requirements of clinical governance and the need for controls assurance, the Committee might consider extending its role to include:

1. Assessing the risks and benefits of introducing new techniques in patient care and monitor the level of training that staff require to provide it.
2. Ensuring that clinicians only practice in fields for which they have been properly accredited.
3. Developing a process that ensures that delegation to junior staff is appropriate for their experience and is made by an explicit and accountable decision.

Discussion of cases can be either in the presence of the clinician involved or in their absence. There are advantages and disadvantages to both methods, although overall the former probably facilitates a more open style of discussion and subsequent recommendation.

The Committee should, through the Medical Director, report to the Chief Executive and the appropriate Trust Board sub-committee charged with litigation issues. The final decision on how to handle claims where external and internal expert advice differ or where other factors predominate, should be taken by the Chief Executive Officer in consultation with the Medical Director, a non-executive director and the Director of Finance, in the light of information from the Trust's lawyers. A decision to settle may be taken on economic grounds despite the ICRC having assessed the case as showing a good standard of care, and in these cases it will be of significant comfort to the individual clinician concerned that they have had the support of their peers. In these difficult situations, particular care should be taken by the Trust and its lawyers to ensure that the professional reputation of the clinician involved remains untarnished.

The Committee should also make clear and specific recommendations for improving clinical process or practice in the light of discussions about the case, and these recommendations should be discussed and agreed with clinical directors, implemented and then tested for compliance by audit after an appropriate interval of time.

The injured patient

The Medical Director and Risk Manager need to have a clear process for dealing with patients injured whilst undergoing care. This will usually include some form of risk management meeting or inquiry to discuss the incident and agreement as to who will counsel the patient and their relatives. Early apology, without necessarily admitting liability, is now generally believed to be the best and most ethical course to pursue. Patients usually want to understand the truth of what happened and to feel that steps have been taken to prevent recurrence. Early, honest, intervention at this stage may often prevent the injury inevitably leading to a legal claim.

Vincent[18] recommends 11 steps for consideration after a patient accident.

1. Believe people who say their treatment has harmed them.
2. Give an early explanation.
3. Decide whether to continue care or refer to another doctor or hospital.
4. Special understanding needed if maintaining the therapeutic relationship.
5. Ask specific questions about emotional trauma.
6. Consider counselling or psychotherapy.
7. Inform patient of changes made after consideration and analysis of the accident.
8. Consider an independent expert report before a complaint or the start of litigation that can be shared with the patient.
9. Consider mediation.
10. Offer compensation.
11. Consider whether the staff response to the accident is indicative of organisational competence in dealing with these difficult situations.

The reaction of staff

Whilst the patient who has been injured in a medical accident needs special attention, so too the staff involved are often seriously affected by the event. It has been reported[19] that doctors faced with a claim experience great distress, worry, anger and frustration and these symptoms are worse when going to trial or being exposed to media coverage. Answering clinical complaints and 'straightforward' visits to the coroner's court can cause considerable anxiety – especially when being questioned by an angry mourning relative. Clinical staff in these positions need support and the Risk Manager should ensure that this is in place and available. Nurses are generally supportive of each other and junior doctors can usually expect their consultant to provide support if not 'take the blame'. Probably the most exposed clinical staff are consultants who often feel isolated and remain silent about the effect of the claim or complaint on them. Some hospitals and the BMA,[20] are now recognising that stress amongst staff needs recognition and support and it has been suggested that staff experiencing a medical accident leading to patient death or injury may benefit from formal debriefing in the same way as those on duty at Hillsborough or Lockerbie.

Conclusion

The introduction of clinical risk management takes many months and there is little to be learnt from the incident database in the first year. Despite requiring a structure in order to function, a clinical risk management programme is really only successful if accompanied by a significant change in culture. All clinical staff need to feel as comfortable about reporting incidents to their manager or the Risk Manager as doctors used to feel about reporting incidents to their defence organisation before Crown Indemnity. An organisation where staff do not fear for their jobs if they make a mistake is likely to be the same organisation that learns lessons from accidents and improves its output as a result.

References

1   Department of Health. *A First Class Service. Quality in the new NHS*. Health Services Circular 1998/113; 1998.
2   The Stationery Office Ltd. 1997 *The New NHS. Modern. Dependable.* London: The Stationery Office, 1997.
3   Morlock LL, Malitz FE. Do hospital risk management programs make a difference?: relationships between risk management programme activities and hospital malpractice claims experience. *Law and Contemporary Problems*; 1991; 54: 1–22.
4   Mills DH, ed. Report on the medical insurance feasibility study. *California Medical Association and California Hospital Association*. San Francisco. Sutter Publications; 1977.
5   Brennan TA, Leape LL, Laird NM, et al. Incidence of adverse events and negligence in hospitalized patients: results of the Harvard medical study I *N Engl J Med*; 1991; 324: 370–77.
6   Wilson RM, Runciman WB, Gibber RW, et al. The Quality in Australian Healthcare Study Med J Aust; 1995; 163: 458–471.
7   Andrews LB, Stocking C, Krizek T, et al. An alternative strategy for studying adverse events in medical care. *Lancet*; 1997; 349: 309–313.
8   Leape LL, Brennan TA, Laird N, et al. The nature of adverse events in hospitalized patients. Results of the Harvard practice study II. *N Engl J Med*; 1991; 324: 377–384.
9   Cooper JB, Newbower RS, Kitz RJ. An analysis of major errors and equipment failures in anaesthetic management; considerations for prevention and detection. *Anaesthesiology*; 1984; 60: 34–42.
10 Gaba DM. Human error in anesthetic mishaps. *Int Anesthesiol Clin*; 1989; 27: 137–147.
11 Runciman WB, Sellen A, Webb RK, et al. Errors, incidents and accidents in anaesthetic practice. *Anaesth Intensive Care*. 1993; 21: 506–519.
12 Reason JT. Understanding adverse events: human factors. In: *Vincent CA ed. Clinical Risk Management*. London: BMJ Publications, 1995.
13 Sheen Mr J, *MV Herald of Free Enterprise*. Report of court No 8074 formal investigation. London: Department of Transport, 1987.
14 Joint Commission on Accreditation of Healthcare Organisations. IMsystem general information. *Oakbrook Terrace IL*: JCAHO, 1995.
15 Maryland Hospital Association. Guidebook for quality indicator data: a continuous improvement model. Lutherville MD: Maryland Hospital Association, 1990.
16 LADD Australia. Early Warning. *Medico-legal News*. 1997; Vol.1: No 3. at p. 2.
17 Knox GE. Obstetrical clinical risk modification; are medical malpractice law suits inevitable? Forum. *Risk Management Foundation*. Harvard: Harvard Medical Institutions Inc Boston 1994; 15: 7–9.
18 Vincent C. Caring for patients harmed by treatment. In: *Vincent CA ed. Clinical Risk Management*. London: BMJ Publications, 1995.
19 Genn H. Supporting staff involved in litigation. In: *Vincent CA ed. Clinical Risk Management*. London: BMJ Publications. 1995.
20 British Medical Association. *Tackling stress in the medical profession*. BMA launches risk management approach. BMA London press release. 30 April 1998.

Appendix 1

Non-specific indicators that have been shown to be associated with claims of negligence.

- Unexpected or trauma related deaths.
- Brain damage or neurological deficit not present on admission.
- Unexpected amputation due to poor outcome of any procedure or treatment.
- Unplanned removal of an organ during surgery.
- More extensive surgery than planned preoperatively.
- Any unplanned return to the operating theatre.
- Operations to repair damage due to an invasive or endoscopic procedure.
- Failure to act upon an imaging or pathology result.
- Pathology/image report to wrong patient.
- Medication error, including infusion pump problems.
- Hospital incurred trauma.
- Equipment failure leading to patient injury.
- Wrong patient or wrong side – surgery or radiology.
- Self-harm or suicide.
- Complication for which patient was not prepared.
- Misdiagnosis.
- Unplanned admission to ICU/HDU.
- Swab/instrument count incorrect at end of procedure.
- Unplanned readmission within 5 days.
- Absent medical notes.

Indicators in obstetrics may include

Infant
- neonatal deaths
- stillbirths
- apgars < 4 at 5 minutes
- any paralysis
- subdural haematoma or tear of falx cerebri
- unanticipated admission to SCBU
- major congenital abnormality first detected at birth
- any fracture
- shoulder dystocia
- meconium aspiration
- fits in nursery within first 48 hours
- iatrogenic injury up to one week after birth
- drug errors
- very low birthweight (? < 900gm)

Mother
- maternal deaths
- transfer to ITU
- convulsions

- major anaesthetic problems, either GA or epidural
- PPH > 1 litre or need for transfusion
- > 30 minutes delay in Caesarean section
- soft tissue injury, 3rd degree tear, ruptured uterus, bladder injury
- injury caused by equipment
- drug errors

Care of the elderly (Courtesy of North Herts NHS Trust)
- Threatening behaviour.
- Damage/loss of property.
- Significant equipment failure.
- Drug errors.
- Failure of follow-up arrangements.
- Failure to act on a clinically significantly abnormal result.
- Falls leading to severe injury or fracture.
- Injury due to equipment.
- Lack of adequate equipment.
- Missing patient.
- Missing medical records.
- Misfiled investigations.
- Pressure sores grade 3 and 4 developing on ward.
- Unable to contact doctor for ill patient.
- Unprofessional behaviour by staff.

Mental health indicators (Courtesy of North Herts NHS Trust)
- Overdose taken by in-patient on unit or while on leave.
- Deliberate self-harm by patient.
- Discovery of an object in patient's possession that could be used for self-harm.
- Discharge against medical advice by a patient not detoxing from alcohol or drugs.
- Absconding from unit.
- Fire-setting in unit.
- Unexpected/sudden death in unit or outside of a patient known to mental health services.
- Patient requesting to see their medical notes.
- Serious physical assault or aggression.
- Discovery of illicit drugs/alcohol on unit.
- Correspondence from solicitor suggesting litigation.
- Injury of unknown origin.
- Drug error.

Paediatric indicators (Courtesy of North Herts NHS Trust)
- Extravasation of iv fluid leading to tissue necrosis.
- Drug dose or fluid prescription error or administration error.
- Failure to recognise the severity of a baby or child's condition or recognise a serious diagnosis.

- Child protection procedures not followed.
- Problems during transportation to a tertiary referral centre.
- Major organisational problems during resuscitation.
- Failure to act on a pathology or imaging result.
- Equipment failure impeding medical provision.
- Unexpected death.
- Delayed diagnosis of severe neonatal hyperbilirubinaemia.
- Sustained hyperoxia grade 3 plus r.o.p. (neonates).
- Delayed diagnosis of important malformations.
- Neonatal ICU – accidental extubation > once in 24 hours.

►8
Claims Management

Myriam Lugon

Since the publication of the Patient's Charter, public expectations have been raised; people have been increasingly aware of their rights[1] and are therefore asking more questions about their care than in the past. The NHS Complaints Procedure was revised to ensure that dissatisfied patients could be provided with timely explanation about their care and in some instances receive an apology;[2] as such over the last two years the number of complaints against hospitals have grown; this has not been associated to a decrease in medical negligence cost. On the contrary the cost and frequency of claims appear to be on the increase with the potential of becoming a financial burden to the NHS.[3] Whether the increased patient awareness of their rights is the cause of the rise in litigation is unclear. Healthcare organisations must, however, minimise clinical risk and ensure that they have in place sound clinical risk management processes and effective mechanism to manage claims promptly; this requires good working relationship with solicitors and a clear understanding of the role of the NHSLA and CNST and their requirements.

The process of managing clinical risk has been described in the previous chapter. Here we will concentrate on describing how Trusts can practically manage claims effectively and use the available clinical expertise to streamline the process, it will not deal with the legal process and framework as it is written in the context of clinical governance requirements;[4] the importance of the relationship between the Trust and their respective solicitors and what can be expected from their services; it will also touch on working with the NHSLA and CNST; particularly in view of the recent publication of the pre-action protocol for the resolution of clinical disputes.[5]

Managing claims effectively – an organisational responsibility

The organisation must give a very high profile to clinical risk and claims management and identify the senior manager whose responsibility this will be, usually a Board member.[6] If at all possible, this should be included in the role definition of the Medical Director; this is not always possible if the Medical Director role is very part time; in these circumstances, it must become the remit of a senior manager with a clinical background, the Director of Nursing. Good working relationship and clear line of communication will need to be established between these two senior managers so that their relevant skills are used to maximum benefit. The lead Director must be supported by an appropriate infrastructure; the size of which will depend on the size and complexity of the organisation. This infrastructure should consist of a Clinical Risk

Manager and if appropriate a separate Claims Manager; these individuals including the lead Director, should be equipped with the relevant skills and should have an understanding of the legal process. These managers will work closely with clinical teams and act as facilitators within those teams so that lessons are learnt from mistakes. To this end, these managers will need to have access to an appropriate IT system helping in the overall management of claims and clinical risk.

In order to manage claims effectively, the organisation must have a sound clinical risk management policy and procedure[7] highlighting roles and responsibilities of all staff from the Chief Executive to the grass root; this should be used as a framework to ensure translation into specialty-specific procedures. These procedures will need to be in place for all high-risk specialties, though over time these must cover comprehensively all clinical activities.

Each specialty needs to identify an individual taking responsibility for monitoring the implementation of the procedure and who will ensure that untoward events, incidents and near misses are reported speedily, investigated and action taken if appropriate. This individual should have a clear line of accountability and be appropriately trained. Close working relationship with all members of the clinical team, the Trust Clinical Risk Manager and/or the Claims Manager if they are different individuals, must be developed; clear line of communication will also need to be established to ensure advice is readily available. This approach rigorously implemented will allow the identification of potential claims at an early stage.

Serious clinical incidents

At times serious clinical incidents may occur; these would include any event resulting in, or with the potential to develop into, serious damage/injury or death of a patient, as an unexpected consequence of clinical care; death or serious injury where foul play is suspected; a number of unexpected/unexplained deaths; a suspicion of a serious error or errors by a member of staff which would give rise to public or professional concerns. This list, however, is by no means exhaustive. Here is a practical example: the diagnosis of acute pancreatitis in a young man in the accident and emergency is missed, the patient is discharged and dies. Such serious clinical incidents often attract media attention. It is therefore important that action is taken early and relatives/patients seen by a senior manager. These should not be left to the common sense of the manager present at the time but enshrined in a clear and explicit process, a serious clinical incident procedure. The procedure should include flow charts defining the role of the staff involved and the action to be taken whatever time of the day or night it is. Box 8.1 describes the process in outline. These incidents are likely to result in relatives seeking compensation from the Trust.

Serious clinical incidents and potential claims identified through the adverse event reporting system must be investigated early when the events surrounding the incidents are still fresh in the mind of the staff involved; and the sequence of events clearly remembered. The Claims Manager will need to be notified immediately so that a copy of the documentation can be secured and a file created identifying the patient's administrative details, the list of staff involved, a chronological summary of the clinical events, worksheets and relevant legal information.[8] Staff must be interviewed and statements

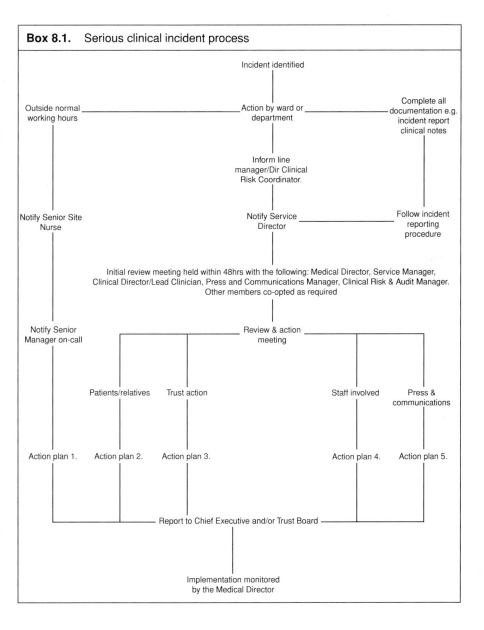

Box 8.1. Serious clinical incident process

Incident identified

Outside normal working hours — Action by ward or department — Complete all documentation e.g. incident report clinical notes

Inform line manager/Dir Clinical Risk Coordinator.

Notify Senior Site Nurse

Notify Service Director — Follow incident reporting procedure

Initial review meeting held within 48hrs with the following: Medical Director, Service Manager, Clinical Director/Lead Clinician, Press and Communications Manager, Clinical Risk & Audit Manager. Other members co-opted as required

Notify Senior Manager on-call

Review & action meeting

Patients/relatives   Trust action   Staff involved   Press & communications

Action plan 1.   Action plan 2.   Action plan 3.   Action plan 4.   Action plan 5.

Report to Chief Executive and/or Trust Board

Implementation monitored by the Medical Director

taken; in case of potential litigation this is best done by the Claims Manager. It is important that they are made aware of the potential for litigation even though the Trust may not have received a letter before action and may not receive one for many months. Up to now statements taken on behalf of legal advisers, are considered privileged information,[9] providing their purpose is to inform solicitors about the case with potential litigation. This may be challenged and in the event, the information gathered will have to be disclosed. Statements must therefore consist of factual information only. The actions of the organisation must be transparent and if negligence is identified during the investigation, this should not be hidden as it will serve no purpose and undoubtedly these facts will come to light during the legal process.

The Claims Manager

Claims must be processed speedily and records of progress monitored and logged. The Claim file as mentioned earlier must be kept up to date and relevant clinical staff kept informed of the different stages the claim is at. This must be the responsibility of the Claims Manager.

The Claims Manager has therefore a pivotal role to play; liaising with the relevant clinical team, the Medical Director, the solicitors, the NHSLA and CNST as appropriate. In England, the majority of trusts have become members of the Clinical Negligence Scheme for Trust, created specifically to protect the Trust against the effect of large claims;[10] this will be discussed in more detail later in this chapter. When joining the scheme, trusts choose their excess and are therefore responsible for the payment in full of claims below the excess. It is therefore beneficial to the organisation if the Claims Manager is able to advise on the organisation's liability and the settlement of small claims in terms of quantum and process; thus ensuring that where negligence and trust liability is established, a quick settlement is achieved to minimise legal costs.

Indeed it is not uncommon for quantum of £5000 to be accompanied by a bill for legal fees of >£25,000; this disparity between costs and damages in medical negligence cases has been highlighted in the Woolf report.[11] A practical guide advising claims managers on the legal process and on good practice for claims management has already been published,[12] the reader should therefore refer to these sources for details that are beyond the scope of this chapter.

Using in house clinical expertise

When claims are being made or when potential claims are identified, it is helpful to have an early view on the appropriateness to settle or defend the claims. In some instances, the decision to settle is easy. Here is such an example: a youngish man undergoes a cataract extraction with lens implant; a month later he develops pain and blurred vision in the eye and presents himself to the A&E Department on a Saturday night and is seen by the on call SHO in ophthalmology; he is examined and referred to the ophthalmic clinic the following Monday; by the Monday morning the wound has broken down and the eye is frankly infected; it is the plaintiff's case that he should have been referred to the specialist hospital on the Saturday. In such cases liability and causation are clear; the costs and damages in such a case could reach £60,000 which could exceed the limit the hospital has agreed with the CNST; the case would therefore need to be referred to the CNST and approval to proceed sought. In many cases, the decision to settle is not so clear cut; expert advice is therefore required.

The Trust has through the staff it employs, access to extensive specialist advice which needs to be harnessed as a cost-effective way of getting expert opinion. By setting up an Incidents and Claims Review Committee (ICRC),[13] the Trust will create a mechanism for taking an early view of the degree to which a plaintiff is correct or incorrect in the assertion of sub-optimal standard of care. Claims will fall into three main categories; those where the standard of care fell short of what is considered acceptable, those where care was of the highest standard and those where there is some degree of uncertainty as to the quality of care delivered.

The ICRC will deal specifically with cases where there is uncertainty about the quality of care and the defensibility of the claims thus providing support to the Trust's lawyers; it will also assist in the Trust's risk management programme in assessing the quality of care provided to patients and making recommendations for changes in clinical or organisational practice. Such a committee needs to be chaired by the Medical Director and consists of senior clinicians respected by their colleagues for their experience and impartiality. Other members should include the Director of Nursing, the Trust Solicitor, the Claims Manager or Legal Affairs Managers and should be serviced by the Clinical Risk Manager. The presence of the Trust's solicitor on the committee is extremely beneficial; it gives him/her the opportunity to gain valuable information on the clinical claims under consideration but also develop the legal knowledge of the clinicians on the committee. The Committee's role is:

1. To review all cases where disclosure of notes has been sought by a plaintiff, particularly difficult cases.
2. To review all cases where the Clinical Risk Management process has identified the potential for litigation.
3. To monitor progress of litigation underway.
4. To make recommendations where changes in practice are required.

The Clinical Risk Manager and Claims Manager meet with the Medical Director to decide on the claims to be considered by the committee. A couple of relevant clinicians are asked to review the appropriate case in depth and present their views at the meeting. The clinicians charged to undertake the review would receive a comprehensive set of information, the other members a summary of the case only. It may be appropriate for the legal adviser to receive more comprehensive information. Each case will be debated in detail before a decision is made.

The decision agreed by the committee will depend on the type of cases presented to them. In circumstances where standards of care are deemed to be poor, consent to an early settlement will be given; the reasons behind the decision must be explicit. The committee should also make explicit recommendations for the changes required in the care process to avoid repetition of the event. In other circumstances, the committee may not be able to reach a decision but requires further information or an external expert opinion. Finally the committee may agree that the care given was of the highest standard and that the case should be defended. Again the reasons behind the decision must be explicit to provide the Clinical Risk Manager and lawyers the opportunity to analyse the committee's rationale and help them prepare a defence. It is important in such cases that the plaintiff's lawyers are notified quickly that having obtained clinical advice, the Trust will not settle. This approach may result in the termination of a dubious claim.

It must, however, be recognised that in some cases the cost of mounting a defence will far outweigh the damages. In such an event, the Trust Medical Director should report the outcome to a panel consisting of the Chief Executive, the Director of

Finance and/or a Non-Executive Director and seek their approval to settle on economical ground. The support for the case from the committee should be communicated to the clinicians involved and the reasons for seeking an early settlement explained. This approach should avoid the discrepancy between costs and damages and ensure that public money is not squandered.

An example of terms of reference for such a committee can be found in Box 8.2. Of course the composition of such committee will vary depending on the type of the Trust (e.g. acute, integrated, community, mental health.)

Box 8.2. Incidents and Claims Review Committee; Terms of reference

The committee will meet on a quarterly basis to review all appropriate new negligence claims against the Trust and is a sub-committee of the Clinical Risk Management Committee.

The following terms of reference applies:

▶ To review all documentation pertaining to new claims including clinical records, witness statements, expert reports and solicitor correspondence if appropriate.

▶ To provide internal expert opinion whenever necessary for the purpose of assisting the Trust in reaching a decision as to liability.

▶ To advise on the procurement of external expert opinion as appropriate.

▶ To identify claims that are suitable for early settlement so that such settlement can be proactively sought.

▶ To identify claims that can be defended and advise the Trust on the approach to be taken.

▶ To monitor the Claims Management Procedure.

▶ To make recommendations for changes in clinical or organisational practice which will improve the quality of care thus preventing recurrence of the event.

▶ To identify clinical risk management issues arising out of claims and advise the Clinical Risk Management Committee.

▶ To ensure strictest confidentiality.

Membership: Medical Director (in the chair), Clinical Risk Manager, Claims or Legal Affairs Manager, Senior Clinicians in relevant specialties, Director of Nursing, Trust Lawyer.

Preventing claims

Healthcare organisations need to manage claims effectively once they have occurred; they also need to concentrate on preventative mechanism. The greatest risk for a hospital is the indiscriminate introduction of new techniques where clinicians experiment without always being equipped with the relevant skills. Whilst organisations need to foster innovations, they need to ensure that developments occur within an explicit framework that will minimise the potential for complications.

The Incidents and Claims Review Committee's role can therefore be extended:

1. To assess the risks and benefits of introducing new techniques in patient care and check the skills and training required in making this technique safe.

2. To set the parameters for the safe introduction of this new technique and monitor its implementation.

3. To ensure clinicians only practice in the field for which they have been properly trained and accredited.

4. To develop a process of delegation to junior medical staff that is safe and appropriate to their skills.

This is the most challenging role for the committee; in effect it would make it the gate-keeper to the introduction of new techniques/interventions. If the benefit of a new technique is based on sound research, the committee will need to concentrate on whether the organisation is able to facilitate this development and whether the staff has the appropriate skills. If its effectiveness is not proven, it may be appropriate to advise the clinician to take part in a randomised controlled trial; the committee would still need to identify the requirement for a safe implementation which includes an assessment of whether the clinician has the necessary skills to undertake this procedure.

Let us say for argument sake, that we are looking at the introduction of laparoscopic cholecystectomy in the local district general hospital. The clinician will need to present his case to the committee answering the following questions:

▶ What support and resources does the implementation of this technique require? Are they available?

▶ Is this technique evidence based?

▶ What are the technical skills required and can he demonstrate that he has acquired the necessary skills to undertake it?

▶ Does the patient consent form highlight the benefits as well as the risks?

▶ How will he monitor the patients' outcomes and complications? Is an audit pro-forma available?

The committee having considered the information presented by the clinician could then agree to the technique being introduced and set the number of procedures to be performed; it will, however, require the clinician to consent the patient himself and undertake a prospective audit to monitor the quality of care and identify complications as they arise. The clinician will be requested to report back to the committee once the number of procedures agreed have been completed.

At the review stage a number of options will be available to the committee:

1. The quality of care was good, no complications were identified. The clinician can continue with the procedure but will be required to continue auditing practice.

2. Organisational issues interfered with the delivery of high quality of care; these will need to be resolved by operational management before continuing with the procedures.

3. There was some deficiency in technical skills which hampered the delivery of optimal care; the clinician will be offered further training in an 'approved' centre where his skills can be brought up to the accepted standard.

4. Too many complications were identified to make this procedure safe; the clinician will thus be required not to proceed further.

This approach is challenging for healthcare organisations; the clinician representatives on the committee must therefore have the confidence of their colleagues and known for their fairness and openness in dealing with difficult issues; in effect they will be challenging 'clinical freedom' and their colleagues' practice. An Incidents and Claims Review Committee undertaking this role will need to develop a clear and explicit process and disseminate it widely. With the increased emphasis on the quality of care and the importance of training and development, healthcare organisation will need to be able to demonstrate that new techniques are introduced safely and undertaken by staff with the appropriate skills. In doing so, they will have proactively attempted to minimise the risk of clinical claims.

Claims and complaints

Complaints will be dealt with in detail in chapter 10. This section will only highlight their important relationship with the claims management process.

The Wilson report 'Being Heard'[14] has resulted in the review of local complaints procedures making it easier for patients to complain about the care they have received. In most instances the patient is satisfied by the explanation of what went wrong coupled with an apology. The investigation of complaints may, however, identify serious clinical mishaps that may give rise to a request for compensation in the future. These must be identified early and the Claims Manager notified so that medical records and statements can be secured and the necessary background work undertaken. It is not always easy to determine the patient's intention when the complaint is received. If the patient is satisfied with the explanation given about his care but feels he is entitled to compensation; this must be dealt with quickly. The complaint must be closed and the Clinical Risk Service asked to progress the request speedily; if the quantum is small, it may not be necessary to involve the Trust's legal adviser; expenses can thus be kept at a minimum.

To ensure that complaints with the potential of becoming claims are identified as early as possible, it would be beneficial for the Complaints Manager and the Clinical Risk and Claims Managers to meet regularly and review the clinical content of complaints. Good working relationship must exist between these different departments and clear and explicit processes in place to avoid duplication of effort and unnecessary delay.

Learning from claims

Any organisation needs to ensure that a climate fostering learning exists and that a non-punitive environment is created. This approach needs to be supported by the Board and Senior Management. All information pertaining to improvement in clinical practice needs to be available and be part of a performance management framework that must be all inclusive. This information should be considered by the various clinical teams and acted upon. Clinical negligence claims data is one set of information to be considered by services alongside clinical incidents reports, clinical claims, clinical effectiveness information, etc. The analyses of the information with the identification of action necessary to improve clinical practice must inform the process of the management team performance review.

The creation of clinical improvement groups[15] at specialty level is a mechanism by which the organisation can ensure that lessons are learnt from past mistakes but also that good practice is recognised. A clinical improvement group must be multidisciplinary, include both managers and senior clinicians, ensure that all 'soft information' pertaining to their specialty is reviewed and actions required identified. The information report needs to examine whether trends can be identified. If events appear to be recurring, the group will need to examine whether standards are adhered to and decide whether an in depth audit is required. They may also need to review the existing standards and develop guidelines if appropriate. This information review may also point to a skills shortage; in which case a decision on the urgency of commissioning the appropriate training programme must be made. Incidents or claims may also recur as a result of defective operational processes; these will therefore need to be addressed in conjunction with the relevant department. The role of this group has been described in more detail in Chapter 3.

Changes required must be accompanied by a clear set of required actions, a lead and time scale for completion must be identified; the individual charged to deliver the actions must be clear about their accountability and the support that is available. The changes in clinical practice or organisational processes must be monitored as part of the performance review process of individual services.

Reporting to the Board

With the introduction of clinical governance, the responsibility for quality will become a statutory function of Chief Executives and Boards. As such they will need to receive and consider the implications of the quality of information presented to them. This has been described in Chapter 3. As far as claims information is concerned, it is important for the Chief Executive and the Board to receive regular update of their contingent liability and keep an eye on trends in claims and their settlements. To this end the quality report must include information on the number of newly reported claims by services/specialties; this may be aggregated to a unit or operational directorate level; categories for reporting will need to be agreed (e.g. unexpected death, misdiagnosis with potential liability). A trend analysis by services/specialties over at least the previous four quarters; and if benchmarking information is available through a network[16] it may be appropriate to compare the type of claims by specialties and examine differences.

This information is clearly sensitive and confidential. Trust Boards are now meeting in public; organisations will therefore need to consider how this is reported to respect staff confidentiality and may thus delegate detailed discussions on these issues to the Clinical Governance Board Sub-Committee described in Chapter 3. The Board must also monitor the implementation of recommendations identified during serious clinical incident investigations and again this may be best discussed in the Clinical Governance Board Sub-Committee.

Ensuring that the Board receives regular information on claims and the Trust contingent liability is only one element of the process of monitoring the quality of care delivered. This information must also be part of performance management of the various clinical services and directorates; thus assuring the Chief Executive and the Board that these issues are taken as seriously as financial probity.

The Trust and its legal advisers

Over 400 Trusts in England are now part of the Clinical Negligence Scheme for Trusts (CNST). The scheme was set up in 1995

> to protect Trusts against the effects of the higher and relatively infrequent clinical negligence claims and to provide a mechanism for smoothing out the financial risk based on principles of mutuality.[17]

Trusts joining the scheme will agree the excess limit (from £10 to £100 K) below which the organisation is responsible for the payment of the claim in full. The CNST has established a comprehensive set of clinical risk management standards with different levels of complexity;[18] if these standards are met by the Trust, a discount on the premium paid is granted. The CNST recently advised its members of changes to the scheme; from the 1 April 1998, the NHSLA is instructing their approved solicitors directly for claims above the Trust agreed limit.[19]

These changes are of significance for Trusts, as they will potentially lose control and influence in the management of their claims; as a result the legal expertise they have built up may be wasted. How Trusts use their legal advisers will very much depend on the excess level chosen. In any case they should seek to minimise expenditure in respect of legal costs and to speed up the litigation process and ensure that legal costs are not spent on cases that are unlikely to proceed. When a claim is received, the first step is to identify whether the claim is above or below the Trust's excess. If the Claims Manager has the skills required to reach a quick and early view on the amount of damages, this can be done in house. In most instances, however, Trusts will not have this expertise available and will need to forward the information to the NHSLA for an assessment.

(a) *Claims below the Trust's excess*: the Claims Manager will, in response to Letters before Action from the plaintiff's solicitors, disclose the case notes, seek statements from Consultant, junior medical staff and other relevant clinicians. The Claims Manager will then seek the views of the Incidents and Claims Review Committee whose membership include the Trust's solicitor, if appropriate; the cases will then be dealt with by the Trust's solicitor depending on whether the case should be settled or not.

(b) *Claims above the Trust's excess*: these claims now need to be reported to the NHSLA who will instruct one of their panel solicitors. If the Trust's solicitors are on the NHSLA approved list, it is important that the Trust approaches the NHSLA to obtain approval to maintain the relationship with their solicitors for claims above the Trust's excess and continue to deal with them directly.

Minimising legal costs

Whatever the level of the claim, minimising legal costs remains an overall imperative and respective Trusts will need to continue carrying out as much preliminary work as possible. It is therefore important that Trusts and their legal advisers agree a plan of action which defines the work necessary on each case and the person responsible for undertaking it. Figure 8.1, prepared by Scrivenger Seabrook, details the relevant steps

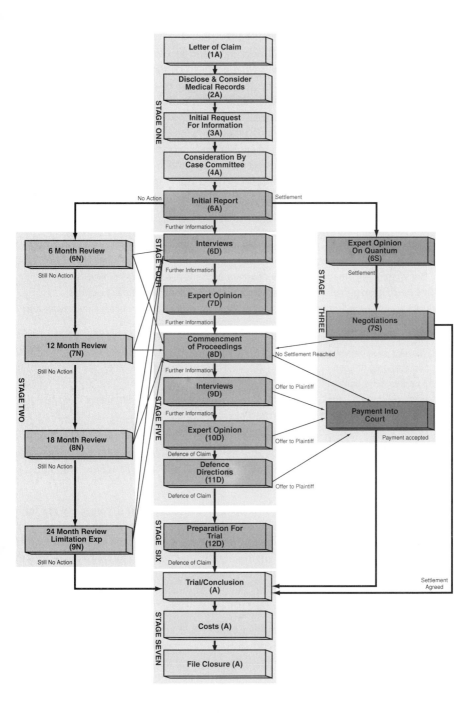

Fig. 8.1. Steps to be followed in Claims Management. Reproduced by permission of Scrivenger Seabrook.

applicable to all claims. The work required for each step will need to be undertaken in a reasonable time scale; the availability of expertise in any Trust will determine what can be undertaken by Trust's staff and what needs to be the responsibility of the legal advisers. Under these circumstances, the Trust will retain some influence on the management of claims whatever the value and ensure that claims are dealt with speedily and the bureaucracy decreased.

The relationship between the Trust and their lawyers is an important one. Managers and lawyers must share and understand each other's expectations and have established clear lines of communication; the lawyers' level of service and commitment must add value to the process.[20] Box 8.3 highlights criteria for working effectively with legal advisers.

Box 8.3. Criteria for effective working

- ▶ Shared goals between legal advisers and healthcare providers.
- ▶ Clear written agreements about management of cases and respective responsibility.
- ▶ One designated person to be contact point both in the legal firm and in hospitals.
- ▶ Direct access by solicitors to the Executive Director responsible for claims if necessary and vice versa.
- ▶ Lawyers must take part in the Incidents and Claims Review Committee.
- ▶ Lawyers must have access to relevant information and relevant clinicians to gain understanding of case.
- ▶ All parties to be cost-conscious.
- ▶ Decisions at the defensibility of a claim must be agreed early by both parties.
- ▶ Confidentiality must be respected at all times.

Scotland, Northern Ireland and Wales have separate arrangements for managing clinical negligence; the funding is top-sliced from the budget made available by Parliament in those regions.

▶ In Wales, Trusts can take part in the All Wales Risk Pool which covers both clinical and non-clinical claims. The Pool is developing clinical risk management standards similar to, but not the same as, the CNST standards; these will be audited by the District Audit function. Hospitals pay a premium into the fund, which is related to the Trust budget; the premiums are increasing to cover both Trust and previous Health Authorities liabilities. Trusts can use the Welsh Office for legal support if they so wish.

▶ In Scotland, the Scottish Central Legal Office acts for NHS Trusts and deals with claims paid out of the Scottish pool; the current level of litigation is very low and there are currently no risk management standards.

▶ In Northern Ireland, the level of litigation is on par with England and paid out of the Common Fund; again there are no formal clinical risk management standard; the Trusts need to tender for their legal services from a list of approved solicitors.

Whatever the system for clinical negligence is, the development of clear and sound process for the management of claims should be a necessary requirement, thus demonstrating a more patient centred approach and greater responsiveness to the public. Clinical Risk Management has been identified as a key element of the clinical governance process, healthcare organisations in the UK will thus be required to develop the appropriate system and ensure sound risk management standards are adhered to.

Working within a national framework – the future

Over the next few years, it is likely that we will see many changes within the medical negligence field. All organisations will need to have proper clinical risk management systems in place and will need to comply with requirements of the civil justice reforms to be implemented in April 1999. This will have implications for healthcare organisations.

The Lord Woolf's report, *Access to Justice*, has an entire section dedicated to medical negligence and litigation.[11] This report highlights deficiencies such as costs often exceeding damages paid, delayed resolution due to the prolonged protracted process; in the main this is believed to be due to delays at the pre-action stage. It also includes many recommendations for healthcare organisations, the General Medical Council and the Legal System (recommendations 187–198).[21] It also highlights the need for patients, healthcare organisations and their respective legal advisers to work more co-operatively and try to resolve clinical disputes rather than proceed with litigation.

As a result of this report, the Clinical Disputes Forum was established in 1997 among others

> to find less adversarial and more cost effective ways of resolving disputes about healthcare and medical treatment.[22]

Their preliminary work has resulted in the publication of a Pre-Action Protocol for the Resolution of Clinical Disputes. This sets out a code of good practice such as the need for appropriate training for staff involved in medical negligence and complaints; the need to deliver care according to accepted standards and routinely monitor it; the need to institute an appropriate incident reporting system; the establishment of clear processes for the storage and retrieval of medical records; the importance of being open with patients and give them timely and accessible information about their care, etc., as well as simple and practical steps to follow when litigation appears likely.[23]

A lot of emphasis has been put on the timeliness of responses and appropriateness of action. The protocol deals with retrieval of health records, letter of claim and the information it must contain (a template has been provided); the suggested format and content of the response from the healthcare providers with a clear time scale. It also touches on expert opinion and the need to consider instructing an expert jointly where appropriate and on alternative approaches to settling disputes. The protocol encourages openness and transparency at a times when the media and some politicians would seem to be increasingly adopting the 'head must roll' approach.[24]

While many trusts now have in place sound clinical risk management systems, it is not standard practice to notify patients and/or their relatives that an untoward/adverse event has occurred except in the case of serious clinical incidents. This duty if imposed, may have consequences for the relationship between patients and clinicians. This protocol will streamline and put some order itno the current process. The practical implications and costs of its implementation will no doubt become clearer as the protocol is used. It is, however, likely that the courts will be given power to enforce its adherence and penalise organisations and their legal advisers in case of non-compliance. The protocol is likely to have an impact on the sequence and time-scale described in Figure 8.1; if adopted as a standard by the CNST, this and further work by the Clinical Disputes Forum will have further implications for the way in which organisations manage their claims in the future. Whether this will curb the escalation of litigation costs remains to be seen.

References

1   The Patient's Charter. *Raising the Standards*. 1992 HPC1. HMSO.
2   EL 95(37) *Acting on Complaints*. Department of Health.
3   National Audit Office. The NHS (England) Summarised Accounts 1995–1996. HC127. London. HMSO. 1997.
4   A First Class Service. *Quality in the New NHS*. Department of Health. Leeds. 1998.
5   The Clinical Disputes Forum. *Pre-Action Protocol for the Resolution of Clinical Disputes*. Clinical Risk. 1998 (4). pp. 139–153.
6   EL (96)11: Clinical Negligence and Personal Injury Litigation. *Claims Handling*. NHSE. 1996.
7   Lugon M. *Developing a Trust Policy and Procedure*. Clinical Risk. 1996 (2): 114–118.
8   Sanderson I. *Anatomy of a Claim*. CNST Review. Autumn 1997. pp. 6–7.
9   Chad-Smith M. *Pro-Active Claims Management*. Healthcare Risk Resource 1997(1) 3: 4–5.
10 Clinical Negligence: proposed creation of a central fund in England. NHS Executive. March 1994.
11 Woolf Rt Hon. Lord. Access to Justice. Final Report to the Lord Chancellor on the Civil Justice in England and Wales. London. HMSO. 1996.
12 Sanderson I. Claims Management: a guide for hospital claims managers. In *Clinical Risk Management*. Ed. Charles Vincent. BMJ Publishing Group. 1995: 492–520.
13 Chad-Smith M. Claims Management: Principles in Practice, Healthcare Risk Resource 1999 (2)3:
14 'Being Heard'. The report of a Review Committee on NHS complaints procedures. Department of Health. 1994.
15 Burke C and Lugon M. *Integrating Clinical Risk and Clinical Audit – moving toward clinical governance*. Healthcare Risk Resource. 1998 (2): 16–18.
16 Merrett H. *Making Connections in Risk Management*. Healthcare Risk Report 1998 (4) 7: 18–19.
17 Sanderson I CNST. A review of its present function. Clinical Risk. 1998 (4): 35–43.
18 Clinical Negligence Scheme for Trusts. Risk Management Standards and Procedures. *Manual Guidance*. April 1996.
19 CNST : Changes to the rules and procedures 1 April 1998. NHSLA. 1998.
20 Jones K. *Managing your Lawyers*. Healthcare Risk Report. 1997, (3) 6: 7–8.
21 Bolger M. *Medical Negligence*. Access to Justice: Analysis of Lord Woolf's Final Report. Healthcare Risk Report 1996 (2) 8: 6–9.
22 Clinical Disputes Forum. *Pre-action Protocol for the Resolution of Clinical Disputes*. Executive summary. Clinical Risk. 1998 (4): 139.
23 Clinical Disputes Forum. *Pre-action Protocol for the Resolution of Clinical Disputes*. Clinical Risk 1998 (4): 139–153.
24 Hopkinson RB. *The protocol: a doctor's view*. Clinical Risk 1998 (4): 154–156.

▶9

Legal Implications of Clinical Governance

Anne-Louise Ferguson

Introduction

From April 1999 all healthcare providers will have to guarantee quality of care under the process of clinical governance incorporating clinical audit, evidence based practice, clinical effectiveness and clinical risk management to ensure that care is satisfactory, consistent and responsive. Every clinician employed by Trusts and Health Authorities will be responsible for the quality of their clinical practice which will be monitored as part of their professional self regulation. Boards of Trusts will be required to produce reports on quality in the same way that financial reports are required. The Chief Executive will carry the ultimate responsibility for ensuring the delivery of a consistently high quality service judged by objective standards.

The purpose of this chapter is to set out what are the existing duties of care within the Health Service, how these are currently treated by the Courts and how the introduction of regulated clinical governance may affect future decisions. It can be assumed that the regulations will be drafted as widely as possible to ensure that the targets set by the Labour Government in the NHS White Paper are achieved but the terms of that statutory instrument are unknown at present and it is not possible to discuss the detailed effects nor the probable sanctions.

Duty of care

It is principle of common law that you must not knowingly cause harm to your neighbour. This principle is applied to the relationship between doctor and patient. When in this century the provision of medical care first involved the state, rather than a personal relationship between doctor and patient, the courts had to resolve the question of whether a state body could owe a patient a duty of care. In *Cassidy* v *Ministry of Health*,[1,10] Denning LJ dealt with the duties of hospital authorities and said:

> In my opinion, authorities who run a hospital, be they local authorities, government boards or any other corporation, are in law under the self same duty as the humblest doctor. Whenever they accept a patient for treatment they must use reasonable care and skills to cure him of his ailment. The hospital authorities cannot, of course, do it by themselves. They have no ears to listen through the stethoscope and no hands to hold the knife. They must do it by the staff they employ and, if their staff are negligent in giving the treatment, they are just as liable for that negligence as is anyone else who employs others to do his duties for him. Is there any possible difference in law,

> I ask, can there be, between hospital authorities who accept a patient for treatment and railway or shipping authorities who accept a passenger for carriage? None whatever. Once they undertake the task, they come under a duty to use care in the doing of it, and that is so whether they do it for reward or not.

However, to date the duty of care imposed by the courts on healthcare providers has not been a general one.

In *Barnett* v *Chelsea and Kensington Hospital Management Committee*[2,10] the facts were that three nightwatchmen attended a hospital casualty department after drinking tea which made them all violently sick, they were seen by a nurse who spoke to the casualty officer on duty about them but he did not attend to examine them; instead giving advice via the nurse. The men left but one subsequently died of arsenic poisoning and the other two were very ill. Neil J in his judgment drew a distinction between a casualty department of a hospital that closes its doors and says no patients can be received, in which case he would by inference have held there was no duty of care, and the facts of this case where the hospital having accepted the men as patients owed them a duty of care not to treat them negligently.

There have been highly publicised legal cases in recent years where a healthcare provider has not agreed to provide an individual with necessary treatment to prolong life because the treatment was too expensive and unlikely to have a long-term effect and the Court has rejected any application to it to force the Health Authority to provide the treatment. In *R* v *Cambridge Health Authority* ex parte B[3] the father of a child suffering acute myeloid leukaemia applied to the Court for judicial review of the Health Authority's decision to accept the clinical judgement of the treating clinicians that further treatment would be of no use in preserving her life. It was argued on the child's behalf that further bone marrow transfusion and treatment with expensive drugs would be of benefit although admittedly only in the very short term. The Court found that it was a rational and logical decision to refuse treatment and even though it was a decision made primarily on the grounds of lack of success, the issue of lack of resources was held to be valid. Resources are finite and the introduction of so-called 'miracle' drugs into the market creates increasing dilemmas to the cash-starved service. It is highly improbable that any sanctions will be applied under new regulations in such cases provided that the healthcare provider demonstrates a reasonable, logical, rationing process.

Duty of care

The patients is owed a duty of care by both the individual doctor and the healthcare provider employing him. If the patient brings a claim alleging that he has received negligent treatment, he may issue proceedings either against the doctor personally, or against the employer: he has a choice. However, it is a general rule at common law that if an employee is negligent in carrying out the terms of his employment, his employer bears the liability for that negligence. In the NHS this has given rise to a formally defined indemnity for NHS covering negligent harm caused to patients or healthy volunteers in the following circumstances:

whenever they are receiving an established treatment, whether or not in accordance with an agreed guideline or protocol; whenever they are receiving a novel or unusual treatment which, in the judgement of the healthcare profession, is appropriate for that particular patient; whenever they are subjects as patients or healthy volunteers of clinical research aimed at benefiting patients now or in the future.[4]

It is important to remember that this indemnity only covers employed staff: those who provide NHS services as independent contractors such as General Practitioners are not so covered and are therefore solely liable in respect of their own negligence or that of their employees. As a result it is essential that they are either insured or indemnified by a medical defence organisation. Clinical governance will also affect general practitioners who are recognised in the government White Paper as having a key role in the new NHS. The standards for these practitioners could simply be those set out by the General Medical Council with the professional standards of support practitioners being also adopted as the quality benchmark.

A fundamental extension of these principles will be introduced in the new statutory requirements for clinical governance, wherein direct liability will also arise where the plaintiffs injury is attributable to some system failure within the organisation. In *Bull* v *Devon AHA*[5] one of the plaintiff's twins was born brain damaged due to the delay in getting the obstetric registrar to attend her. The defendant health authority maintained maternity services on two sites and the system for calling the registrar between sites to deliver the babies had broken down. This was considered to be negligence but not medical negligence because no individual had breached their duty of care to the patient or the babies but the system operated by the hospital was not of an acceptable standard to deliver appropriate care.

Individual responsibility

The advent of clinical governance may bring individual responsibility for such systems failures and with it appropriate sanction. If statutory responsibility for the delivery of a quality service falls on the Chief Executive of a Trust or Health Authority then such decisions as the appointment of staff and the delegation of work to that staff are also ultimately his responsibility. Already in existence is the principle of corporate responsibility of a hospital or health authority being directly liable to the patient in negligence rather than the clinicians who treated the patient where the hospital trust had employed staff who were insufficiently experienced or frankly incompetent and, therefore, unable to cope with the requirements of the post to which they had been appointed. In *Wilsher* v *Essex Health Authority*[6] a junior doctor mistakenly inserted a catheter into an umbilical vein for arterial blood gas sampling. The senior registrar did not recognise the mistake then compounded the mistake by repeating the error when the catheter was replaced. The premature baby suffered near total blindness due to oversaturation of oxygen causing retrolental fibroplasia. The Court of Appeal found that

a Health Authority which so conducts its hospital that it fails to provide doctors of sufficient skill and experience to give the treatment offered at the hospital may be directly liable in negligence to the patient . . . I can see no reason why, in principle, the health authority should not be so liable if its organisation is at fault.

In such circumstances it would not be the inexperienced or overtired doctor or nurse who would be sued for negligence but the employer who would be directly liable. This case also raises the vexed question of doctors working unreasonably long hours which results in lack of sleep which has been shown to dramatically affect performance. Although the newly introduced Working Time Directive restricting working hours to forty eight per week does specifically exclude junior doctors it is suggested that a failure of a hospital Trust board to recognise the affect this may have on quality is of direct relevance to the principles of clinical governance.

It will be necessary to identify quickly those members of staff who consistently perform badly and take steps to remedy the problem either by referral to the individual's professional body or by offering retraining or, when appropriate, terminating their employment. Clear guidelines will be necessary to ensure that problems are recognised and reported early in order to prevent falls in standards or significant medical negligence claims which are extremely costly to the Trusts. This is a difficult area to enforce but clinical governance demands the delivery of consistency of standard and it will not be acceptable for one directorate to be seen to be failing due to one poor performer. This direct liability for staff performance may be extended by the new statutory requirement to encompass non-clinical staff who have a direct contribution to the delivery of a quality service. The Chief Executive of any employing healthcare provider must ensure a very efficient recruitment and training structure to avoid leaving poor performers in post in order to avoid both censure and penalty if the statute so provides. The recent Bristol case will be the influencing factor in this aspect of the chief executive's duty of care.

In some circumstances individual clinicians and health service providers may also owe a duty of care to a third party, such as to a relative, arising out of the treatment given to the patient but the establishment of such duties is more complicated. In a recent decision the Scottish Court has awarded the sum of five thousand pounds to the father of a Downs Syndrome baby in a case brought by the couple against the hospital. Unusually the court held that the hospital owed a duty of care to both parents rather than only to the patient, the mother, who was negligently treated when the hospital failed to offer an amniocentesis which would have shown that the baby was damaged; so depriving the mother of the opportunity to have an abortion and avoid the shock of giving birth to a handicapped child.

Risk management

In England the National Health Service Litigation Authority set up by statute in 1996 has implemented risk management standards which all member trusts of the Clinical Negligence Scheme for Trusts must work towards achieving by certain given dates. In Wales, the Welsh Risk Pool has implemented similar, although slightly more stringent, standards also to be achieved by stages within a certain length of time. Those risk management standards and their compliance by trusts is to be audited annually and it would be open to a plaintiff in a medical negligence action to seek disclosure of the audit process in order to provide support to a claim that the failure to achieve certain standards required under the statute governing the provision of quality care resulted in breach of that duty.

Documentation of every kind which is generated in the management of a healthcare provider is deemed discoverable, or in other words, discloseable to a plaintiff who sues it if the documentation did not come into existence solely for the purpose of litigation. All audit documentation, guidelines and protocols, minutes of audit meetings, data generated under Health and Safety Regulations, estates agendae may all, in principle, be called for once litigation has been commenced. It is a requirement of both NHSLA and the Welsh Risk Pool that a senior member of a Trust or Health Authority Board must be the accountable officer in respect of risk management policy and there is, therefore, the unedifying prospect for that officer that he or she may be called to give evidence at court in any action for negligence in which a systems failure due to poor risk management practice is alleged to be the cause of damage to the patient.

At present the standard of care required to be shown by an individual doctor is that referred to as the 'Bolam' principle.[7] The facts, which are little known and never referred to now because they are not as important as the principle the case established, were that the plaintiff suffered from clinical depression and the decision was made to use electroconvulsive therapy which was a fairly new treatment in the 1950s and not widely used. Treatment required the passing of an electric current through the patient's brain to induce a fit but understandably had a number of side effects including causing bone fractures because of the jerking of the patient during the treatment. When the plaintiff underwent the treatment he was held down by nurses holding only his chin, this was insufficient to prevent his body from convulsing and he suffered serious pelvic injuries. Evidence was given that alternative methods of restraint included the use of relaxant drugs and much more rigid restraint. However, it was recognised then and is still recognised that medicine is an art, not a science and different schools of thought regarding the best use of different treatments can coexist. McNair J in Bolam said:

> A doctor is not guilty of negligence if he has acted in accordance with the practice accepted as proper by a responsible body of medical men skilled in that particular art.

This is the 'Bolam' principle and it has been applied by courts in medical negligence cases ever since. Although there have been discussions about the application of this principle in all cases, the House of Lords reaffirmed the application of the 'Bolam' test in *Bolitho* v *City and Hackney Health Authority*.[8] This case, however, qualified the 'Bolam' principle in order to give back the courts some influence in the judicial process by proposing that it was not sufficient that a practice was followed by a group of skilled medical men but went further to say that that practice must be reasonable and supported in logic. Thus the court would be able to judge whether practice which might cause harm to a patient should not be regarded as acceptable simply because several medical experts accept it as common practice.

Evidence based medicine

The increasing interest and research into evidence based medicine is likely to have a further impact on the 'Bolam' principle. The philosophy behind evidence based medicine is that it should be more a science than an art as has previously been the case. Each treatment or intervention will be based on the knowledge of previous successes with evidence of a high probability of success rather than on a trial and error basis. If it is known that a certain condition responds to a certain combination of the most expensive drugs, coupled with surgery requiring intensive therapy care afterwards then it will not be sufficient to try one of the drugs in isolation or to adopt a wait and see policy, as might presently be the case. The issue with regard to clinical governance is that this removes some of the freedom which presently exists for clinicians and has resource implications which will need to be addressed by the Chief Executive and the board of the healthcare provider.

It has been rare for Chief Executives of either Health Authorities or Trusts to regard clinical effectiveness as their own responsibility but under the standards of clinical governance this will become a requirement. If there is not direct accountability at board level for the clinical effectiveness of treatments offered and for the adoption of evidence based practice and it can be demonstrated that their own decision making processes lack evidence and logic, it is unlikely that clinical effectiveness will be achieved in a directorate. One of the chief difficulties of evidence based medicine is that there is insufficient pooling of information between clinicians and service providers. The introduction in the future of a comprehensive Information Technology system for the National Health Service may begin to address this shortcoming. However, it will become a major responsibility of the Medical Director of each hospital to ensure that clear and well promulgated guidelines and protocols in respect of evidence based practices are in place and are easily accessible, in order to be effective.

Guidelines and protocols[9]

One question often asked of lawyers is 'are there any differences between protocols and guidelines and how they are treated by law?'. The answer is that strictly speaking, they are not recognised in law where there is no mandate and no sanction. However, guidelines are drawn up in order to be followed. A guideline can be no stronger than a proposal which may 'guide' in any given situation, be simple advice or recommendation. However, where clinical guidelines do exist to provide guidance on specific circumstances to clinicians it is necessary to follow those guidelines because to fail to do so may result in a practice which falls below the standard of care deemed 'responsible and appropriate' by those clinicians who would be deemed by the court to be a 'reasonable body of medical opinion' (Bolam).

It could be argued that guidelines are only as good as the author or authors who produced them and as such can be superseded by new or different guidelines. Suffice to say that where a guideline is recognised to be in place and generally followed, departure from such guidelines may lead to both censure in court and, worse, a judicial finding that the care given which fails to be in accordance with those guidelines is negligent. Guidelines will not ever be used as a substitute for expert evidence in court. This is because they cannot be subject to cross examination unless the author of those guidelines is present to speak to them. However, the converse is also true, guidelines which are felt by a clinician to be unreasonable and illogical and which are, therefore, not followed are unlikely to be applied by the court if it accepts that medical opinion as reasonable and logical.

Where regulations and guidelines are issued by statutory bodies these are more likely to be followed by the courts and will take rather more argument to challenge. In the future all guidelines relating to matters concerning clinical governance must be robust enough to be used throughout a Trust unless specific to a certain area of care. Presently a significant area of risk lies with the lack of clarity of procedures and intentions of interacting different agencies such as the primary and secondary health providers and between different hospitals or hospital and social services. Traditionally an area which has been overlooked; clinical governance will demand clear, unambiguous and closely followed guidelines if a high quality service is to be achieved. Failure to implement such a system may result in litigation which is likely to require discovery to the court of defective guidelines or protocols.

Are protocols different from guidelines? The dictionary definition of 'protocol' is 'a record of an agreement'. It could be argued, therefore, that it is has slightly less force than a guideline but has its place within the process of clinical audit to reduce the possibility of maverick practices which may affect the delivery of quality care. The supervision of compliance with clinical governance directives is likely to fall to the new Commission for Health Improvement described in the Government's NHS White Paper. It is too early to sit in judgement on whether or not the imposition of clinical governance will achieve all its aims to improve quality and remove regional variations in standards. However, the proposals in relation to the Commission do not provide for it to have an overall role in the co-ordination of all the existing institutions responsible for monitoring of clinical effectiveness, quality and responsiveness of healthcare providers, such as the Ombudsman, complaints bodies, the General Medical Council etc. For the moment there is no indication of just what sanctions the Commission may have in order to give it teeth and it is not, as yet, known what sort of sanctions may be introduced under the new statutory requirement for the delivery of quality care and speculation at this stage is unhelpful.

Pre action protocol for the resolution of clinical disputes

Lord Woolf, Master of the Rolls reviewed the civil justice system and found it sorely in need of reform in order to provide wider and fairer access to justice. During the course of his review he recommended that the pre-litigation process was an inefficient way to deal with complaints made by consumers of the Health Service. Consequently the Clinical Disputes Forum was set up in 1997 to include many individuals involved in all aspects of medico-legal matters to find more effective ways of resolving such disputes. The basic premise being that there has been a breakdown of trust between the healthcare providers and the consumers, the former believing that often a complaint is unjustified but its investigation is time consuming, and the latter who believe that there are 'cover ups' and that doctors and nurses 'close ranks' in the event of an 'error'.

The purpose of the Protocol is to encourage a climate of openness when something has gone wrong during the course of a patient's treatment, or the patient is dissatisfied with either treatment or outcome. This is a direct reflection of the requirements for clinical governance. It also addresses the delays which presently occur in dealing with complaints and claims. The Protocol makes general recommendations about training of the staff who must handle complaints and claims. It also makes specific reference to adverse incident reporting systems which will be key tools in the improvement in and maintenance of quality standards under clinical governance. The Protocol will be effective in April 1999 at the same time as the civil justice system begins its new age. The principles are the same and equally well-meaning; that all disputes are managed as quickly, efficiently and as openly as possible.

For the healthcare provider and its staff it will be necessary to treat claims as an absolute priority in order that an investigation and explanation, and where appropriate, an apology are provided within three months of receipt of a letter of claim. Penalties will be applied if a response is too slow or if the claimant issues proceedings too hastily before other avenues of dispute resolution have been explored. A similar protocol has been drawn up to provide guidance for the claims in personal injury actions.

The present two tier court system where both the High and the County Court each operated by its own discrete set of rules will be merged and there will be one new set of rules for the new court. These will be applied much more strictly in order that timetables are adhered to and parties in breach of the rules will be subject to sanctions, such as payment of significant levels of interest on damages suggested but not agreed to. The intention is that the judiciary will become extremely efficient case managers using information technology to ensure that courts are not subject to over-booking or lacunae. The process of litigation itself will be speeded up, reducing costs and ensuring satisfactory outcomes.

Conclusion

The law relating to the duty of care owed to patients by individual clinicians and subsequently by their employing healthcare bodies has been developed by the courts under the principles of common law over the past fifty years. Little in the way of statutory regulation has been introduced on the grounds that it has not been required for the protection of the consumers of the health service. It is now recognised that inconsistency in the standards of care have not nor cannot be satisfactorily addressed by the doctors and nurses governing bodies alone because in very many cases the fault lies less with an individual's breach of duty of care and more with a failure in the system to ensure a high enough standard of care. The statutory regulations governing the principles of clinical governance are intended to overcome this failure but it remains to be seen whether the provisions of the statute are far-reaching enough and whether the sanctions are sufficient to ensure compliance.

References

1   *Cassidy* v *Ministry of health* [1951] 2KB343.
2   *Barnett* v *Chelsea and Kensington Hospital Management Committee* [1968] 1 All ER1268.
3   *R* v *Cambridge Health Authority* ex parte B (a minor) 1995 23 BMLR1CA.
4   Health Circular NHS Indemnity – Arrangements for Negligence Claims in the NHS, October 1996.
5   *Bull* v *Devon AHA* [1993] 4MED LR117.
6   *Wilsher* v *Essex Health Authority* [1986] 3All ER.
7   *Bolam* v *Friern Hospital Management Committee* [1957] 1 WLR582.
8   *Bolitho* v *City and Hackney Health Authority* [1997] 4 All ER.
9   Hurwitz B *The Authority and Legal Standing of Clinical Standards and Practice Guidelines*. In Effective Clinical Practice. Miles A and Lugon M. (Eds) Blackwell Science, Oxford, 1996.

►10

Learning from Complaints

Susan Hobbs

Introduction

In general terms most patients, their families, friends and carers have considerable trust in the services that the National Health Service (NHS), provides. The majority of patients experience high quality care but where they perceive a drop in standards they have a right to be heard and for their complaints to be dealt with promptly, efficiently and politely.

So why do people complain about the health service? It is widely accepted that the NHS is an incredibly complex organisation. In total it employs over one million staff. It treats more and more people year on year, providing more and more complex care, pushing back the very frontiers of science and technology; yet many consumers of a service that is considered internationally by many as the epitome of good practice, remain dissatisfied. Arguably the very nature and complexity of such a service would suggest that it was never, or ever will be, a perfect service; so what has changed recently to develop a more consumer focus on the delivery of health services?

In the past 20 years the public sector in virtually all industrialised nations has changed dramatically. Long held assumptions about the role and function of the public sector have been removed to be replaced by ideas largely borrowed from private sector business and performance measures, strategic and business planning, the importance of management information, increased accountability and the pressures of the internal market. Add to that shift the continuous and very public pattern and pace of change, which has set the agenda for the NHS since the 1990 reforms. In particular the advent of the Patient's Charter, the very essence of which was to widen choice and to make the health service more responsive to patients' needs. All have further raised public expectations of a service that is arguably unable to meet the level of quality to which it aspires. The public and media interest in all things clinical, whether fact or fiction (and sometimes it is difficult to tell the difference), have all changed our overall perceptions of the health service. Indeed the consumers expectations of the public sector, fuelled for some by increasing wealth and for others – the old, the sick and the poor – by increasing needs, continue to rise and be disappointed.

What triggers complaints?

We know that people complain for different reasons. The so named '*Wilson*' report[1] stressed that all complainants want to be taken seriously. The committee commented that

> Complainants can face an uphill struggle when using the NHS Complaints Procedures, firstly in making their views known and, secondly in receiving the sort of response they would wish for.

There is no doubt that complainants want their views to be acknowledged. They want an explanation. They also want the individual or the organisation they hold responsible to be prepared to take action and to be told what has been done to put matters right. To maintain public confidence in the NHS it is essential that all complaints be investigated thoroughly and without bias.

Complainants, particularly if they are patients, often feel uneasy about voicing their concerns in the first place. Many genuinely feel that by complaining about any aspect of treatment and care they are jeopardising any further treatment that may be required. They are not usually in a powerful position, they feel vulnerable, and the ability of the organisation to respond positively and quickly will become the benchmark for the resolution of the issue, others often feel that the whole process is an exercise in damage limitation.

A simple apology may be what the complainant really wants. The apology should be unconditional, if this is not forthcoming the complainant is less likely to be satisfied. Experience tells us that all too often a failure or unwillingness to apologise at an early stage is the reason for complaints proceeding further through the system than is really necessary or appropriate. Recent research found that most complainants only wanted an apology and to be convinced that the same thing would not happen to others.

One particular report stated that in 70% of incidents progression to litigation would not have happened if there were an early apology.[2] It would appear that it is better to seek out possible dissatisfactions than let the situation escalate to anger or a formal complaint. This puts staff on the defensive, initiates worries about legal liability if a mistake is admitted and draws the battle lines. Many complaints' officers and others who investigate complaints are fearful of the risk of litigation. If this is a real possibility a clear policy must be agreed which allows clinical and managerial staff to give full and honest explanations to patients and relatives on humanitarian and clinical grounds, even at the risk of ensuing litigation. When something has gone wrong taking an active stance in communicating with patients and carers so that early restorative action can be initiated, before they complain, can only be beneficial. As many patients sue partly because they want an explanation,[3,4] this is probably a sound financial policy as well as a humane one.

Equally some complainants may also want action which has a more direct bearing on the nature of the care provided to them, such as faster or additional treatment, or financial compensation. However, even in cases relating to clinical judgement complainants do not always have financial compensation as a primary goal. Some who go on to take legal action do so simply because other goals are not being met.

Sadly complaints about the NHS are viewed by some staff as being an irritating intrusion, some colleagues are often immediately defensive and resistant to any investigation taking place into their own clinical practice even to the point of obstruction.

Changing policies

Reference was made earlier to the Wilson report. This came about as a result of a thorough and far reaching review of complaints procedures that the government of the day announced in 1993 in response to mounting criticism of the previous complaints procedure. The shortcomings of previous systems were widely described as follows:

▶ Complainants faced an uphill struggle in making their views known and in receiving the sort of response they would wish for.

▶ People did not know who to complain to.

▶ There were too many different procedures and people involved.

▶ NHS procedures were seen to be often ineffective in meeting complainants objectives and would often increase dissatisfaction.

▶ Very few organisations had any visible written information about the complaints system.

To address these issues a committee chaired by Professor Alan Wilson, Vice Chancellor of Leeds University, was established by the then Secretary of State. Its objective was to review the procedures available for the making and handling of complaints by NHS patients and their families in the United Kingdom and the costs and benefits of finding alternatives to current procedures. The committee reviewed practice in the NHS as well as examples of different approaches in both the public and private sectors in Britain and in the health service of other countries. The Committee recommended that the following principles should be incorporated into new NHS complaints procedures:

▶ responsiveness

▶ quality enhancement

▶ cost effectiveness

▶ accessibility

▶ impartiality

▶ simplicity

▶ speed

▶ confidentiality

▶ accountability.

The report published in May 1994 recommended major changes based on three principles:

▶ That there should be a common system for complaints covering all NHS services.

▶ That the system should be geared to the complainants concerns and that disciplinary action should be kept separate.

▶ That there should be a two stage approach, the first in-house, starting where the complaint arises; the second an investigation by an independent panel.

Acting on Complaints, became the revised policy document and proposals for the new NHS complaints procedure in England were published in March 1995. Full guidance on the implementation of the agreed new NHS complaints procedure was introduced in March 1996,[5] and NHS Trusts, Health Authorities, Family Health Service Authorities and General Practitioners were expected to design and operate their own complaints procedures, using the guidance document as a framework, while adhering to the legal requirements of the appropriate Directions and Regulations.

The key objectives for the new procedure reinforced the guiding principles, and all NHS organisations were expected to demonstrate and reinforce compliance. The monitoring of complaints procedures, and in particular the attainment of compliance to targets has become part of the contract monitoring arrangements. From a commissioning perspective and in the absence of formal accreditation systems new complaints procedures should be seen to be enforceable through existing contracting mechanisms as part of quality monitoring.

Complaints management and customer care training

Throughout this decade much emphasis has been placed upon enabling staff to respond positively to patients' and carers' concerns, questions and criticisms, and to improve information. Previously customer care training had in the main been absent in the public sector, and a huge cultural shift has had to be effected in many NHS organisations for its place in the training portfolio to be accepted and understood. Learning how to handle difficult situations, including potential complainants, is an integral part of customer care training and arguably should be mandatory for every new member of staff who has a role which brings him or her into direct contact with patients and carers. In addition there should be specific training for a wide range of staff in dealing with dissatisfied customers. This training should be considered to be as important as any other and as such should be planned and funded as part of the organisational development and training programme.

Locally, following a survey of medical students a one-day programme is being developed jointly between the College of Medicine and the Trust. The programme will cover many aspects of risk management, including scenario planning and the handling of complaints. Non-attendance is not an option. From a recent review of complaints we certainly need to accept that empathy, sympathy and the ability to admit mistakes are attributes that many clinical and managerial colleagues need to acquire and maintain. Support and even counselling for colleagues directly involved in disturbing or injurious incidents should also be available if considered appropriate.

Customer care training – guiding principles

Complaints should not be seen as the responsibility of the customer relations department only. Everyone in the organisation needs to contribute to:

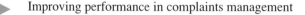 Handling them effectively

Improving performance in complaints management

Accepting and applying the lessons learned from them.

Handling complaints properly is an important part of good customer care. It shows that you:

- Listen to your users views

- Learn from your mistakes

- Are continually trying to improve your service.

Access to the complaints procedure must be simple and the language used easily understood, this will:

- Encourage complaints and compliments by advertising your procedures and making them easy to use.

- Inform all your users about your service standards and how to complain if you do not meet them.

- Make it clear to the public that you welcome complaints and comments and that you will use the information to improve your services.

- Make provision for users who have special needs, for example those with a reading, hearing or language difficulty.

- Enable you to regularly audit your procedures.

A good idea which you can use to support ward and departmental staff is to compile a 'survival kit' on handling complaints. This will:

- Encourage front line staff to 'own' complaints.

- Give staff immediate access to clear written procedures that focus on sorting out complaints quickly.

But remember to:

- Consult staff and users when drawing up and revising complaints procedures.

- Make sure that the procedures are fair to staff and users, and that information is treated as confidential.

- Recognise the importance of good communication skills when recruiting and training staff who handle complaints.

- Make sure that all staff know about the procedures and receive training.

- Draw up a menu of remedies and make sure that staff and users understand the options open to complainants, including the role of the Ombudsman.

- Support your staff which in turn will improve their commitment to handling complaints properly.

- Get the basics right:

  - listen carefully

  - investigate properly.

Getting and using results from complaints

> Record all complaints and analyse them regularly to understand users views and the improvements they want to see.

> Establish an effective complaints monitoring group, preferably with membership from the Community Health Council, or other patients' representatives.

> Collate regular reports for management teams, looking at trends and changes in the pattern of complaints which may arise as a result of changes in service delivery or configuration.

> Publish information at least once a year on:

>> the number and type of complaints

>> how quickly they were dealt with

>> user's satisfaction, and actions taken as a result

>> pass information from complaints monitoring to policy makers

>> take advantage of new information technology

>> subject complaints monitoring to peer review.

Local resolution

The Department of Health places great emphasis on resolving complaints as quickly as possible. This may be through an informed response by a frontline practitioner or through speedy and open investigation and conciliation by other staff empowered to deal with complaints. The mandatory process of Local Resolution is therefore a comprehensive entity in its own right and not simply a run up to an Independent Review. The Medical Defence Union (MDU) also supports strongly the principle of Local Resolution of complaints. Anecdotal evidence suggests that properly handled local procedures will resolve around 75% of grievances. Speed, sympathy and a willingness to listen may be all that is necessary.

Complaints and risk management

No organisation can devote sufficient resources to eliminate all risks. Things will inevitably go wrong. Just as aircraft will crash, banks will be defrauded and oil tankers will sink, healthcare professionals will give incorrect treatment or a lack of care.

Risk management is an organisational response to a need to reduce errors and their costs. In most NHS Trusts risk management is now regarded as an integral component of the general management process, and not an optional extra. It has clear links with quality improvement programmes, but more than with other quality assurance initiatives it places a special emphasis on the costs and consequences of poor quality care. Risk management is fundamentally a particular approach to improving the quality of care, which places special emphasis on occasions in which patients are harmed or disturbed by their treatment or care. Thus a coherent, comprehensive and accessible complaints management policy should be accepted as an essential component of the overall risk management strategy. The prompt management of complaints, avoidance of litigation or the early settlement of damages should benefit both the complainant and Trusts.

The interplay of human and organisational factors that result in errors is complex.[6] Adverse occurrences in patient care are not uncommon,[7] and although only a small proportion of these result in significant damage or distress and even fewer in litigation, much unnecessary distress arises from failure to deal honestly and effectively with such events as they occur. Often patients are denied what they need most, an explanation of what happened, and when this fails to materialise they are forced into lodging a formal complaint. The complaints procedure may be protracted, even when it does not proceed beyond the local system. The cost of dealing with even minor deficiencies in care, in terms of patient or carer distress can escalate wildly. Dealing promptly and effectively with complaints is part of risk management. To do this an open approach to complaints management and their antecedents – adverse events and mishaps – is needed.

Case studies

It is always valuable to look at other organisations' complaints case histories and learn from them. The following are all taken from one Trust's complaints tracking system during one year. The names used are fictitious but the scenarios described, the issues identified and the actions taken as a result are real – all make for salutary reading. All have changed clinical and managerial practice.

● Case study 1

Mr J was a 78-year-old gentleman who was admitted under the care of a General Physician with a respiratory infection in January 1997. He responded to the treatment given, but developed acute retention of urine for which he required catheterisation. He was transferred to a surgical ward and subsequently scheduled for a Prostatectomy under spinal anaesthesia on 13 February. The operation was successful, following which the patient was in good spirits. His blood pressure and body temperature were low, but he appeared to be making a good recovery. During the period between 14 February and 20 February the patient was left without medical care, or at least documented medical care, for at least three days.

The patient subsequently died on 20 February and his relatives believed that his death was preventable. A full internal investigation was undertaken and the recommendations made were actioned.

Issues

▶ Communication.

▶ Referral procedures.

▶ Documentation.

▶ Accountability for decision making.

Action taken

The case was thoroughly investigated by a small panel and both medical teams were seen. An audit of medical and nursing notes was undertaken and recommendations for improvements made. The introduction of bed management has considerably improved the situation in relation to knowing where patients are, in particular when transfers are made out of normal hours or at the weekend. Communication between Consultant Medical Staff who either initiate or accept referrals has been improved through the use of protocols. The family was contacted after the investigation by the Medical Director outlining the lessons that had been learned.

● Case study 2

A young woman was admitted to deliver a child. The child was born with a deformity to an upper limb. The family agreed that as this was a distressing deformity and that they did not wish the facts to be made public, they would tell people in their own time. They were then further distressed to learn that at least two of their neighbours knew of the defect within two days of the birth. One neighbour even came to the grandparent's house to offer condolences. At the same time a relative of the family was employed by the hospital in another clinical area. The family alleged that this person had discovered the information easily and had passed it on to the individuals concerned. It was then further complicated by the fact that the complainants felt that the matter had not been dealt with properly and that they had been refused an interview to discuss the matter further. They also wanted disciplinary action taken against the staff member concerned and had great difficulty in separating out the two issues. This case remains unresolved as far as the family is concerned, even though it has gone to an Independent Review Panel and was not fully upheld.

Issues

▶ Confidentiality.

▶ Access to medical notes.

▶ Abuse of position (staff).

▶ Delays in complaints management system.

Action taken

No disciplinary action was taken as a result of the investigation, but all staff have been reminded of their privileged position in relation to confidential and sensitive information. The induction programme for all staff has been strengthened. Medical records have reviewed and improved tracer systems for notes. Notes are no longer left outside the patient's door in the maternity unit. A review of complaints management has been undertaken and the changes implemented as a result were supported by the Trust Board.

● **Case study 3**

Mrs B was admitted to a District General Hospital as an emergency admission with severe airway obstruction, secondary to a large benign goitre. She was known to be asthmatic but had been in reasonable health before this obstruction episode. On admission her trachea was intubated by an Anaesthetist and she was stabilised in the Intensive Care Unit whilst her lungs recovered from the effects of the crisis which had occurred around the admission. She remained intubated until a tracheostomy was performed, and after that a tracheostomy tube maintained the patency of her airway. She was later transferred to an ENT ward when considered to be stable. The tracheostomy tube was initially of a Portex type, but, despite this tube, her airway became blocked, once again necessitating oro-tracheal intubation. This was promptly converted to tracheal intubation with a special tracheal tube. Some four weeks from the emergency admission Mrs B was transferred as an elective transfer to a teaching hospital for further management of her goitre. She was transferred by ambulance to an ENT ward, but was by this time largely self-caring, walking to the ward toilet as required. Tracheostomy care was being provided by the nursing staff with a regimen that included 2 hourly suction. Suction was planned for 0015, but at 2350, the patient was found to be in respiratory difficulty by a trained nurse. Subsequently the patient suffered a cardio-respiratory arrest during which she incurred hypoxic/ischaemic brain damage. There were issues raised after the event which included the integrity of the equipment available, the arrest procedure itself and the training and responsiveness of clinical and administrative staff. There seems little doubt that the incident significantly contributed to her death some two months later.

Issues

▶ Environmental safety post transfer.

▶ Management of cardiac arrest.

▶ Communication.

▶ Resuscitation equipment.

▶ Staff training.

Action taken

This case was presented to the Risk Management Committee and key members were asked to discuss the issues and bring back an action plan. Whilst it was considered that the patient was transferred to a safe environment it was felt that the staffing level and skill mix could have been enhanced, even though the patient was essentially self-caring. Cardiac arrest procedures have been reviewed and additional training agreed. Equipment has been updated and associated training agreed for staff.

● **Case study 4**

Mr B was admitted for elective coronary artery surgery. He had a history of stable angina and had suffered one myocardial infarction. The surgery went well and the immediate postoperative phase was uneventful and his care was stepped down from intensive care to high dependency. During the second postoperative day he was noted to have an irregular

---

heartbeat. This dysrythmia and others lasted for seven days. They were treated with various medications and procedures including carotid artery massage and elective cardioversion. On the twelfth postoperative day he was noted to have increasing abdominal distension. He was referred to a general surgeon and underwent an emergency laparotomy. At operation his bowel was found to be ischaemic and perforated. During the next 24 hours he required two further operations including a splenectomy, subsequently his condition deteriorated and he died. His wife complained about many aspects of his care. The complaint was investigated thoroughly, but she and her family remained dissatisfied and a request was made for an independent review.

Issues

▶ Delays in diagnosis and treatment.

▶ Documentation.

▶ Communication by staff.

▶ Postoperative care management.

▶ Delays in complaints procedures.

▶ Transfer procedures.

▶ Referral procedures.

▶ Supervision of junior staff.

▶ Relatives and decision-making.

Action taken

The report from the Independent Review Panel suggested that the Trust review its procedures to ensure that patients referred to Consultants are seen by the Consultant who will be responsible for their treatment and care. Further the Panel asked that both patients and relatives be more closely involved in discussions about treatment, procedures and possible outcomes, and for medical staff to be clear about who will perform the procedure. Inter-hospital referral procedures were identified as being in need of review. The issue of the supervision of specialist registrars in the operating theatre was clarified with the Royal College of Surgeons and reinforced by the Medical Director. The complaints management procedures were already under review at the time and the recommendations following the internal review have been implemented.

● **Case study 5**

Miss H was a 54-year-old lady with learning disabilities who was admitted for elective neurosurgery to remove a pituitary tumour. The surgery went well and her postoperative recovery was uneventful, the main concern being to ensure optimal endocrinological function. This was managed through an appropriate referral to a specialist physician. On the fifth postoperative day the patient was visited by a relative, who took the patient out of the ward for a walk. Whilst the patient was out of the ward she fell and was brought back to the ward, having apparently sustained an injury to her upper arm. The patient was later seen by a junior doctor, but was not x-rayed initially. When she was x-rayed she was transferred to another hospital, within the same Trust, to the care of the Trauma Unit. The relatives were not informed of the transfer at the time. During her time on the trauma unit the patient became very unwell, and she was subsequently transferred back to the original hospital and readmitted to a high dependency unit under the care of the endocrinology team. Her condition was stabilised and she was eventually moved back to a medical ward for a further programme of rehabilitation. Sadly her recovery was poor after this event and after a further transfer to a hospital nearer her home she died a few months later. A relative kept a detailed diary of events throughout the patient's hospitalisation, the details of which make for stark reading set against the issues raised.

Issues

▶ Lack of care.

▶ Communication failures.

▶ Lost medical notes.

▶ Care planning.

Action taken

A multi-disciplinary meeting has been held with the relatives and the questions that they have raised have been dealt with honestly and openly. Whilst statements from clinical staff have been taken it is very difficult to be able to refute the allegations in the light of the continuing absence of the patient's medical records. The case remains open.

All of the case studies had an element of poor communication within them, all could have been handled better and could possibly have been managed more effectively and positively for the Trust and the complainants alike at an earlier stage. It seems clear that there are occasions when we have to acknowledge fault, accept responsibility, without admitting liability and work harder to ensure that we do learn from our mistakes through the sharing of case studies. The Trust in question now actively reviews cases periodically in a multi-disciplinary setting, after which the cases are used at Directorate level as a learning opportunity.

In addition to the specific actions demanded as a result of the investigation of individual complaints other actions have been taken to learn from complaints based upon an analysis of the top four classifications. The most common complaints surround diagnosis and treatment and some of the issues raised have been identified within the case studies. The following, in order, are classifications of the next highest numbers of complaints together with some action points.

Staff attitudes

Directorate training packages have been devised based on real cases that have been anonymised. The Health Service Commissioner's epitomes are also used specifically to draw out problems, which occur as a result of poor staff attitudes. Individual staff members are also invited to attend meetings with complainants and to give feedback to colleagues. Customer care training is now applied across the staff groups.

Poor communication

An emphasis is placed on staff maintaining good communication both written and verbal through induction programmes and in house training. This is an ongoing problem, which despite the best efforts continues to be a regular problem with complainants.

Waiting times

Individual Directorates are made aware of specific areas of concern through the formal managerial monitoring arrangements, contracting discussions and the requirement to furnish commissioners with key information set against agreed performance indicators.

Complaints management – what have we learnt so far?

The number of complaints continues to grow and the Health Service Commissioners Office (HSC), expect a 10% rise in their workload year on year. During 1998/99 the HSC has established working procedures for clinical investigations and is now open to receiving complaints about clinical judgement and the actions of Family Health Services Authorities will now be under the jurisdiction of the HSC. There is also a steady increase in the requests for Independent Reviews which further underlines both the public's insistence on being heard and the need to work harder on local resolution.

The complaints also appear to be becoming more complex. Complaints have a host of causes, poor training, poor communication, wrong information, high stress levels, defensiveness in managing criticism, staff perceptions, lack of priority, inappropriate management. Consequently if you look at the complaints which are generated over a period of time, for any organisation, the number received will vary – but they will be centred round an average, and it is the average that counts. Managers and committees who monitor complaints levels as a measure of performance must understand that variations from month to month are significant only if they deviate significantly, or there is a persistent trend. If this happens then there is a specific cause which will need to be investigated and an action plan developed.

As was described earlier it can be demonstrated that the two most common causes of increasing numbers of complaints since 1990 have been the launch of the Patient's Charter and the implementation of the recommendations of the Wilson report, both of which increased the accessibility and awareness for complainants. To have interpreted these events as a sign that there was an overall decrease in performance across the health service could have proved demoralising and led to excessively negative investigations. Such actions can foster a blame culture that discourages reports of 'near misses'. Quite simply the NHS needs its complaints procedure to:

- satisfy complainants
- enhance the reputation of its service
- avoid protracted correspondence
- avoid unnecessary litigation

- use complaints as a means of improving services

- be fair to staff

- maintain a balance between treating staff appropriately and maintaining proper accountability for their actions.

Conclusions

Complaints can be used positively in several ways. They can provide an opportunity for providers to see themselves and their service as others see them and to identify the issues, which concern users. Most importantly, complaints can allow for rectifying a past mistake and enabling services to be put right for the future. A well-handled complaint can increase a patient's trust in doctors, nurses, other healthcare staff and managers. Finally complaints can enable the identification of adverse events, which might otherwise go undetected; they may also be the 'tip of the iceberg', the indicator of a bigger or deeper problem, which can be investigated at an early stage. They can act as an early warning system for legal claims and, if properly categorised, contextualised, recorded, and analysed, can identify areas for quality improvement plans.

Our aims must be to reduce the chances of a catastrophe to negligible levels and to deal effectively with the less severe but more common incidents that form the basis of most complaints. In trying to do this, there is always a temptation to concentrate on tightening policies and procedures rather than examining the organisational culture. This is because these are the tangible controls that can be audited and measured and that in turn restore public confidence. Clearly these actions have their proper place but, managing risk is as much a matter of values, leadership, organisational culture and effective communications as it is about good management systems – and this must be reflected in the way complaints are handled.

Complaints are often quoted as being the source of ideas for quality improvement programmes, but there are many facets to this and one important question is, does your organisation appreciate the potential of the complaints it receives? Understanding the implications of your complaints is central to the actions that you and your organisation take to improve quality, the messages that are given to all staff and the organisational culture that supports risk management. Complaints can provide input to support clinical audit, risk management and quality initiatives. Genuine partnerships between patients, their families and advocates and NHS staff can result.

The best of all worlds is a partnership with patients, which looks at complaints as a valued tool for improved quality – not a measure of Quality Improvement. Complaints should play a part in improving standards by initiating systematic review of incidents and triggering action to avoid future problems.[8] Effective handling of complaints should include learning from the situation and preventing recurrence, in line with recent developments in clinical risk management.

A study published in July 1994,[9] showed that complainants want changes to be made as a result of their experiences. The result from this study highlighted several key issues that required recognition and action if the quality 'loop' was to be closed and similar incidents avoided in future. The study found that most incidents stemmed from incidents that led to significant clinical consequences and distress. In many instances deterioration in the patient's clinical condition had led to additional treatment and longer stays in hospital. Secondly clinical complaints are seldom about an error of clinical judgement alone but are often about staff insensitivity and poor communication. Thirdly, the way the complaint was handled compounded the difficulties and intensified the distress or dissatisfaction that had led to the complaint in the first place. Finally complainants often emphasise the need for more involvement in decision making in relation to their condition and treatment and about being kept better informed about progress and problems. Simple enough, but we are back to the basics of providing adequate information, being effective communicators and accepting our roles as partners in care.

Footnote

'A customer is the most important visitor on our premises. He is not dependent on us – we are dependent on him. He is not an interruption of our work, he is the purpose of it. He is not an outsider on our business – he is part of it. We are not doing him a favour by serving him – he is doing us a favour by giving us the opportunity to do so.' **Mahatma Gandhi**

References

1   Wilson Committee. *Being Heard.* The report of a review committee on NHS complaints procedures. London. Department of Health, 1994.
2   Kent P. *Apologies are the best insurance.* Letter. Health Service Journal, 21/3/91; 10.
3   Simanowitz A. Standards, attitudes and accountability in the medical profession *Lancet* 1985; ii: 546.
4   Simanowitz A. *Accountability.* In: Vincent CA, Ennis M and Audley RJ, Eds, *Medical accidents.* Oxford. Oxford University Press, 1993; 209–221.
5   NHS Executive. *Complaints, Listening, Acting, Improving.* Department of Health, March 1996.
6   Reason JT. Understanding adverse events; human factors. *Quality in Health Care* 1995; 4: 80–89.
7   Bennett J and Walshe K. Occurrence screening as a method of audit. *British Medical Journal* 1990; 300: 1248–1251.
8   Bark P et al. Clinical complaints: a means of improving the quality of care. *Quality in Health Care* 1994; 3: 123–132.
9   Bark P et al. Clinical complaints: a means of improving the quality of care. *Quality in Health Care* 1994; 3: 123–132.

▶11

Clinical Governance and Education and Training

Tony Weight, Kate Phipps, Neil Jackson

Introduction

The definition of clinical governance uses the term 'framework' and stresses the accountability of NHS organisations for improving quality[1] and allowing 'excellence in clinical care'[2] to flourish. Explicit in this definition is managerial accountability for high quality services but equally implicit is ensuring that the provision of clinical care by professional staff is excellent. Where is this excellence to come from? How will professional staff be guaranteed to possess the knowledge, skills and attitudes necessary to provide this excellent service?

This is where the appropriateness and effectiveness of their education and training will play a crucial part. It is the education and training received by professional staff that will determine to a very large extent the quality of service provided. It is the application of their education and training in a clinical setting that is fundamental.

The term education and training is used widely. By it, is meant the learning events that a healthcare professional will experience from the time they enter a programme to qualify as a professional (e.g. doctor, nurse, occupational therapist), right up until the time they retire from working as a professional in the NHS. Very nearly cradle to grave, and certainly learning that lasts a working lifetime.

Clinical governance is a new term but not a new concept. Many of the building blocks for clinical governance at the organisational level are already in place.

Effective clinical governance needs to be underpinned and supported by education and training of healthcare professionals that is relevant, up-to-date, flexible in its delivery and meets the needs of the individual professional as well as the needs of the organisation in which they work. Only if education and training measures up to the above criteria will healthcare staff be able to contribute to high quality services and excellent clinical care. Without it clinical governance will not work.

Education and training – levels of analysis

If education and training is so important to the effective implementation of clinical governance, then it is necessary to understand the main characteristics of the education and training arrangements currently operating within the NHS. The analysis can then give some key messages for the future management of education and training and by implication clinical governance.

It would be inaccurate and misleading to see the education and training impact on clinical governance as being determined solely by the effectiveness and appropriateness at an individual professional level. Three more levels of analysis are needed.

▶ First, at the level of the clinical team. This could be in a trust or in a general practice. Working effectively in a clinical team has long been accepted as a major determinant of high quality care. Interdependency between different professions has made team-working essential.

▶ Second, the focus for the implementation of clinical governance is at the local or organisation level (i.e. NHS Trust and Primary Care Group). An organisational development plan will be required to support the implementation of clinical governance throughout an organisation by education and training programmes which will seek to change behaviour and attitudes as well as the setting up of organisation wide procedures, and monitoring systems.

▶ Third, the impact of the national levy based system of education and training investment cannot be overlooked. The three educational levies that make up the national education and training system exert a huge influence on individual, professional teams and the organisation. In terms of financial investment the application of a total sum approaching £2 billion nationally must be understood.

The education and training system

The term education and training system is used here as part of a three system approach to healthcare, the other two systems being service and research and development. It is the complex interaction of the three systems that makes up the dynamic of the provision of healthcare.

The three education and training levies – Service Increment for Teaching (SIFT), Medical and Dental Education Levy (MADEL) and Non-Medical Education and Training Levy (NMET) are all derived from Health Authority allocations. SIFT is a levy which funds the additional costs to the NHS of supporting the clinical teaching of undergraduate medical students. It is not a payment for teaching but a subsidy designed to provide a level playing field between NHS Trusts. MADEL covers part of the basic salaries of doctors in training and the local costs for the facilities for post-graduate medical and dental education (i.e. post-graduate centres and libraries as well as the cost of study leave).[3] NMET covers the education costs of the education and training of professions other than doctors and dentists and its funding is distributed via contracts between universities which provide pre-registration or undergraduate programmes, student bursaries and some limited education salary support to Trusts.

Each levy is therefore different in concept and operation and they are kept separate by a no virement budget rule. In some regional offices, co-ordination of the three levies at the point of use is made possible where accountability is rested in a Director of Education and Training. The three levies make up a national education 'system' which is managed regionally or locally and ultimately impacts in some way on all professionals working in the NHS and on their education and training. A basic appreciation and understanding of the levy based systems is essential to analyse how it will influence the implementation of clinical governance at a local level.

Education and Training is sometimes seen as a learning event that takes place away from work and is somehow divorced and remote from it. A significant part of the operation of the education 'system' described above is university-based but an equally significant part is the practical application of that academic learning. Both at undergraduate or pre-registration level and at post-graduate or post-registration level, NHS Trusts and General Practices are significant providers of education and training through the practical training they provide, commonly referred to as a clinical placement.

Established infrastructure

This means that all NHS Trusts and many General Practices have an established infrastructure for providing practical training for students who are either studying for a first qualification or who are maybe undertaking practical training to further their professional knowledge and skills. This is best demonstrated by the long period of education and training a 'junior' doctor will undertake once they have qualified as a doctor. The MADEL Levy will ensure salary and other support in an established post at Trust level that enables continuous education and training and work to happen side-by-side. The same is true for nurses pursuing further professional education and training. The NMET levy will provide the tuition fees to the university. In all probability, it will be the nurse's employer (i.e. the NHS Trust which will provide the practical work-based experience). The same would apply to a doctor undertaking GP vocational training in a General Practice.

NHS employers are therefore an integral part of the education system and contribute hugely to the education and training activity financed through the levy-based system.

Education and Training needs to be continuous to enable a healthcare professional to carry out their duties to a high standard. Great emphasis is put upon the requirement for effective Continuing Professional Development (CPD) arrangements at an individual and team level and CPD is defined as 'a process of lifelong learning for all individuals and teams which meet the needs of patients, and delivers the health outcomes and health priorities of the NHS and enables professionals to expand and fulfil their potential'.[4]

CPD as defined above needs to be an important part of the education and training system but crucially its operation needs to be sensitive to individual and organisation needs and must be managed and applied locally. One potential dilemma is the matching of the individual or team's needs with the wider service needs. These two are not always the same and attempting to reconcile both can lead to conflict where service needs do not meet professional aspirations.

Wide spread debate

The current levy-based education and training system invests heavily in education and training which comes within the definition of CPD. The challenge is ensuring that future investment in CPD is relevant, appropriate and achieves the twin objectives of meeting service as well as individual need. There is wide spread debate about the extent to which some of the levy-based investment is currently attaining those objectives, particularly in terms of equity of access to all health care professionals and its appropriateness. One of the main criticisms has been the extent to which current education and training investment is education-led rather than employer-led and is therefore not sensitive or appropriate to local service needs. Because of the all pervasive nature of the levy-based system, investment in MADEL and NMET needs to be rigorously reviewed to try and ensure that education and training programmes which come into the CPD definition can meet the challenges set out in *A first class service. Quality in the NHS*.

Education and Training Consortia were established in 1998 and are a recent important development in the Education and Training system. Composed of Health Authorities, Trusts, GP representatives and representatives from the voluntary, independent and local authorities sectors, their role is to plan and commission education and training for those professional groups funded through the NMET levy. They are geographically based and are a collective of employers aiming to forecast the current and future requirements of their professional workforce and produce an annual education and training investment plan which supports the healthcare strategy plans and service provision plans of its constituent members. Although their remit is the NMET levy, it is anticipated that their workforce-planning role will expand to take in medical and dental workforce planning, both at secondary and primary care level. Education consortia provide a focal point in the education and training system and over time have the potential to develop as the arena where truly integrated workforce planning and development can take place.

They have an important role in commissioning education from education providers and determine annually the number of student training places on undergraduate or pre-registration education and training programmes. From April 1998 a majority of the consortia in the NHS in England became fully responsible for budget, commissioning, and workforce planning.

Initiatives and innovation

These consortia are able to plan with a relative degree of freedom and significantly have the opportunity to pursue initiatives and innovation in education and training provision by the judicious use of development funds. These funds are being used in some consortia to pursue different modes of delivery of CPD programmes, multi-disciplinary and multi-professional programmes and responding to national policy developments by supporting the development needs of the newly emerging primary care groups. Opportunities have also been taken to widen the access to CPD programmes to professions that traditionally have not had access to NMET levy funds.

The post-graduate deanery plays an important commissioning role for Post-Graduate Medical and Dental Education (PGMDE). PGMDE is funded by the MADEL levy and the post-graduate deans set standards, against which training is purchased, determine where training should take place and allocate training resources between trusts.

The Deanery is closely involved in the regulation of pre-registration house officer training and arrangements for flexible training for doctors in training with family or other personal commitments and the GP Vocational Training Scheme and Specialist Training Committees. They work in close co-operation with the Royal Colleges and Staff Training Committees (STCs) in carrying out their role. The Deans also maintain close links with their local education and training consortia and by these links, contribute to the development of an integrated approach to workforce planning.[5]

Universities as providers of academic education and training, are essential components of the education and training system. They are heavily involved in the arrangements for undergraduate medical and dental training and therefore are linked closely to the operation of SIFT, working closely with post-graduate deans for PGMDE. They also enter into education funding contracts with education consortia for the provision of programmes for the professional groups covered by the NMET levy. The developing relationship between organisations in the NHS and Universities is extremely important in ensuring the current and future quality of education and training provision. It has become increasingly necessary to stress the nature of the relationship as one of partnership and collaboration and for the NHS and universities to mutually recognise and understand each other's perspective on issues affecting education and training in the NHS, particularly in relation to funding by the NMET levy. For some universities the level of funds invested via education and training contracts, amounts to a significant percentage of their total income. The NHS is a major purchaser of education and training in the university sector and therefore needs to assure itself that the investment is effective, appropriate, of a high standard and represents value for money.

Professional and Statutory Bodies

The education and training system within the NHS is not only managed internally. The role of universities has been described. Of equal importance are the roles and responsibilities carried out by Professional and Statutory Bodies. Their primary role is to ensure the quality of education and training programmes and that the trainees or students once qualified or registered, are safe to practise their particular profession.

For medicine and dentistry this role is undertaken by the Royal Colleges. They devise their authority by Royal Charter, laid before Privy Council and are the bodies accountable for assuring the quality of practice in the craft or specialty for which they are responsible. They set standards for post-graduate education and training that must be attained and define the competencies that trainees must achieve. They also confirm that appropriate medical training has been completed satisfactorily by an individual trainee. This allows the registration as a specialist of the individual by the General Medical Council. For Nursing, Midwifery and Health Visiting, the United Kingdom Central Council for Nursing, Midwifery and Health Visiting carries out this role. It is supported by four national boards, the English National Board (ENB) being the one linked to the NHS in England. Amongst its statutory duties laid down by the Nurses, Midwives, and Health Visitors Act of 1979, are determining and establishing the kind, content and standard of programmes of education and training with which the National

Boards must comply. The ENB will approve institutions that provide education and training programmes to enable individuals to qualify for registration as a nurse, midwife or health visitor. It also has power, like the Royal Colleges for Medicine and Dentistry, to withdraw training approval status from an institution (i.e. a university or an NHS Trust).[6]

A large number of the other professions are covered by the Professions Supplementary to Medicine Act 1960, which established a council to regulate the initial training and fitness to practise of all the following professions; chiropodists, dieticians, medical laboratory scientific officers, occupational therapists, orthoptists, physiotherapists, radiographers, art therapists and prosthetists and orthotists. Each profession has its own board responsible for approving training courses and training institutions and qualifications as well as maintaining a register of persons qualified in their respective profession. Each board approves new or revalidated courses. For the professions of clinical scientists, clinical psychologists, pharmacists and speech and language therapists, these have professional boards similar to those of the CPSM.[7]

The role of professional and statutory bodies in supporting CPD is recognised as:

▶ influencing or setting the standards of clinical practice

▶ promoting professional self-regulation

▶ supporting audit of practice and relating it to learning needs

▶ promoting life long learning amongst professional staff.[8]

Each employer must take account of other influences including its membership and role within local education and training consortia and its relations with the post-graduate deanery. It must also take account of how the education and training system interacts with, and is affected by, the related systems of service and research and development.

Organisational education and training

NHS Trusts, future Primary Care Trusts and Primary Care Groups will be the main organisational vehicles by which clinical governance will be established and implemented. It is at this organisational level that commitment to, and support for clinical governance must be sustained. Education and training at organisational level can be seen as a means of achieving this, by helping to make a cultural change and encouraging a much better partnership between professionals and managers.

The following encapsulates the organisational requirements; clinical governance requires partnerships within healthcare teams, between health professionals (including academic staff) and managers, between individuals and the organisation in which they work and between the NHS, patients and the public.[9]

Clearly systems and processes will need to be set up to support the introduction of clinical governance but that alone will not be enough. Leadership by management but also by professionals will be a key factor in assisting cultural change within an organisation. There may well be a need to identify, develop and support professional leaders locally. This inevitably will involve a mix of different professionals who will require an organisation culture which supports multi-disciplinary working and learning. The other important factor is to try and see the implementation of clinical governance as part of a supportive and positive organisational climate rather than being seen merely as 'weeding out' poorly performing professionals. Cultural change and resulting changes in attitudes will take time to be achieved and all levels of the organisation must be targeted. In the same way that individual professional employees will need development plans so organisations themselves must have development plans with clear measurable targets, and a culture which encourages evaluation and feedback. They will form part of a yearly plan for clinical governance, which will form the basis of clinical directorate plans, as well as being the basis for an annual report from the NHS Trust Board.

Whilst NHS Trusts have had the time to implement corporate governance and may be assumed to be better placed to get a head start in implementing clinical governance, organisations in primary care pose particular problems because of the rapidly changing nature of primary care organisations and the relatively small size of general practices.

Primary care groups

The preoccupation with issues concerning the setting up of primary care groups will mean that the timetable for implementation will be longer. Already newly-established primary care groups have been given a requirement to identify a 'lead' person for clinical governance. The role of the health authority in assisting primary healthcare professionals to embrace the philosophy of clinical governance will be important.

Organisational values towards the individual and their Continuing Professional Development (CPD) will need to change. Organisations must recognise and support the need for individuals to have dedicated time to enhance their knowledge and skills and work towards more equitable access for that time and the education and training programmes required. They must also address and recognise the need to reconcile differences between organisational needs and individual needs where these exist. They will not always be complementary and compromise on occasions will be necessary. In the fast changing world of the NHS, professionals do not always see service developments and priorities as their own developments and priorities.

Education and training at the organisational level can be seen in two different but related dimensions.

▶ First, the education and training needed to generate cultural change, knowledge and awareness of the concept of clinical governance and the supporting infrastructure of systems and process for its implementation.

▶ Second, the education and training needed to sustain and develop continuously the individual professional's level of knowledge and skill which will ultimately determine the quality of patient care provided.

Whether in primary or secondary care, professionals working together to provide high quality care have always been seen as absolutely essential. Whilst each professional brings their unique core knowledge and skills to a care programme, in many situations the opportunity and the ability to work together makes the real difference in effective healthcare provision.

Team education and training

The importance of effective team-working is not necessarily reflected in the education and training arrangements favoured by individual professionals. Certainly at pre-registration or undergraduate level, common core programmes for two or more professional groups are the exception rather than the rule, even though common areas within the curriculum can be identified. Education and training within the same institution for different professional groups does not guarantee a joint or common approach either.

The current education and training system seems to militate against such developments. Fear of dilution of the profession's status or uniqueness could be part of the issue, though there are many professionals who would see such developments as welcome and an obvious endorsement of the team-working concept.

If not at pre-registration or undergraduate level, then for CPD there should be greater opportunities at the organisational level for learning together. Again the current position is patchy. It could be argued that the development of clinical governance will help the movement towards a greater frequency of the instances of multi-disciplinary learning. An organisation that is progressive in its approach to clinical governance will be emphasising the values of professionals learning together to complement their working together and must be providing the environment and supportive culture within which this can take place.

Multi-disciplinary education

The move towards a philosophy of multi-disciplinary education and training is now accepted as a priority but two important points need to be stressed.

▶ First, that as much as there is a need to develop multi-disciplinary and multi-professional approaches to education and training, there will always be instances where uni-professional education and training is also required to maintain and update the knowledge and skills of a professional group. A balance between the two is required and must be accepted. A mixed economy of approaches to education and training at post-registration or post-graduate level is essential.

▶ Second, there needs to be a much greater evidence-based approach to support the move to multi-professional learning programmes. There does not appear to be sufficient evidence available that multi-disciplinary learning works. Support for it is now unquestioned but the evidence of its effectiveness remains largely hidden.

The final issue for clinical governance in teams is that of team leadership. As has already been stated the need to identify and support professional leaders will be vital in developing clinical governance.

The professional leaders will need to be practising clinicians in order to have credibility with peers and there will no doubt be challenges to the view that the professional leaders should in most cases be medical!

Individual education and training

Integrated care for patients will rely on models of training and education that give staff a clear understanding of how their own roles fit with those of others within both the health and social care professions.

This quote[10] neatly sums up many of the issues facing the individual professional in taking their share of responsibility for clinical governance.

Professionals have a link to the patient, a need to understand their own particular role within the organisation or the team and the need to be continuously identifying their personal development needs. The effectiveness of an individual professional's contribution to high quality care will be a function of many things including:

▶ Their own motivation and willingness to learn and realise their potential.

▶ A supportive manager who identifies the learning needs with the individual and agrees a personal development plan.

▶ An employer that recognises the need for personal development and encourages it.

▶ Being able to access funds and training programmes through an effective framework of CPD locally, linked to the education and training system.

▶ A realisation that personal development needs will not always match the needs of the organisation in which they work.

▶ A cycle of personal development planning which starts with assessment of need, moves on to planning, then implementation and finally evaluation.[11]

This model recognises the continuous cyclical process of CPD and therefore reinforces the notion of 'lifelong learning'.

Personal development planning

Personal development planning will be an important part of the CPD cycle and is likely to be in two distinct parts. The first will be a detailed set of work objectives, mutually agreed with the individual's manager which will cover a period of time, normally a year. They will be supported by success criteria (how will the individual know that the objective has been achieved), deadlines for achieving the objective and dates for reviewing progress in meeting those objectives. The process will need to be flexible so that objectives can change in scope, nature and extent in response to changing work circumstances and situations. This will require clarity in the work role of the individual, clarity in their duties and be linked to a set of competencies identified with effective levels of work performance. A competency based approach to help define effective work performance, together with defining work roles by the use of occupational standards has grown in influence within the NHS in the last five years. This approach in any newly developed system of personal development planning is likely to be used by some NHS employers.

The second distinctive part to a personal development planning system will be a training and development plan, linked to the work objectives. Again, this will be mutually agreed and will detail training and development objectives, the approach to be used to achieve that objective (e.g. training course, on the job training, shadowing or coaching or other learning events, criteria to demonstrate improvement in that particular area and how the training and development helps to achieve the work objectives). It will not always be the case that an identified training and development objective is directly related to a work objective and in extreme cases may only demonstrate a tenuous link. This is because in personal development planning, longer term personal aims are just as important as the immediate work objectives and local management and employers need to be sensitive to and supportive of future career aspirations as a legitimate part of a personal development planning process. Demanding targets have been set for employers to have training and development plans in place for the majority of health professional staff by April 2000.[12]

Commissioning education to meet identified needs

Personal development plans based on individual as well as organisational need will be brought together into a team or directorate plan. This then is put in priority order, costed and forms part of an overall organisational education and training plan which is again put into priority order and costed. This will enable the local education and training consortia, and post-graduate deanery, to focus more effectively on commissioning education to meet identified needs.

The dilemma of matching individual training and development needs to organisational needs can be demonstrated by considering the position of the individual in terms of three elements of their fitness. For a professional who is newly-qualified, they will have proved their fitness for award (i.e. the academic level of attainment awarded by the education provider by examination). They will have satisfied the requirements of the professional and/or statutory body, which validated the education and training programme and therefore have demonstrated fitness for practice (i.e. demonstrated their ability to practise safely as a professional). The requirements placed upon them in their job by their new NHS employer can be met by them demonstrating fitness for purpose. This can equally apply to an experienced professional. Fitness for award, practice and purpose are all linked together, but it is the potential mismatch between practice and purpose that can generate tensions between the individual, their professional and/or statutory body and employer. Service development needs as articulated by an employer in terms of job role and duties do not always match expectations of the safe practitioner. This tension is sometimes translated into personal development plans where needs as perceived by the individual are at odds with organisational needs. One solution to this difficulty is for employers through collectives such as education consortia to state more explicitly what fitness for purpose means and how this is to be incorporated within curricula at undergraduate and post-graduate level. There can then be less of a gap between the perceptions from different stakeholders in the education and training system of fitness for practice and fitness for purpose.

> The government will continue to work with the professions, the NHS and patient representative groups to strengthen the existing systems of self-regulation by ensuring they are open, responsive and publicly accountable.[13]

The reference to strengthening self-regulation acknowledges the established practice within the NHS that professionals have the right to set their own standards of discipline, conduct and professional practice. This self-regulation is separate from sanctions that can and may be imposed upon an individual professional employee by their employer. Ultimately this can mean the loss of a job. The essential difference to self-regulation is that professionals falling below set standards can endanger their right to practise their profession.

Self-regulation arrangements must have credibility and have the confidence of patients as well as other staff in the NHS. Quality of care is so important that any arrangements for self-regulation must demonstrate the ability to deal with serious lapses in that quality when they have occurred. Education and training at an individual level should be seen as one significant contribution to maintaining the level of knowledge and skill necessary for a professional to continue to practise safely and to a high level of performance.

Key messages

This chapter has tried to demonstrate a significant connection between clinical governance and education and training at the level of the education and training system, the organisation, the team and the individual. In analysing these levels, there are a number of key messages that must be considered in the implementation of clinical governance. These are:

▶ The crucial importance of effective and appropriate education and training that derives from the needs of the professional workforce, which is in turn providing a relevant, modern and high quality service. The link between education and training service provision and quality of care is clearly made. The link being the job to be done and how well it is done.

▶ The need for education and training at all levels to be responsive to a rapidly changing healthcare environment.

▶ The need to understand the levy-based education and training system and to take advantage of it to support innovation in education and training.

▶ The need for organisations in particular to connect with education and training consortia and the post-graduate deaneries, both of which are key parts of the education system, and which can help the organisation and the individual to 'plug in' to the education and training system.

▶ The need for a mixed economy approach to support multi-professional and uni-professional education and training.

▶ The need to develop evidence based approach to multi-disciplinary education and training.

▶ The need to use the knowledge of the education and training system to reform current arrangements for CPD to make it more equitable, more accessible and part of a staff strategy at the organisational level.

▶ The need to reconcile fitness for award, practice and purpose.

▶ The need for cultural change at organisation level which produces support and encouragement for personal development.

▶ The requirement for personal development needs to be matched as far as is possible with organisation development needs, but accepting that this is not always going to be possible.

▶ The requirement that a competency based approach complemented by occupation standards is a growing influence in defining level of job performance.

▶ That the links between clinical governance and education and training will continue to evolve and be part of an iterative process.

▶ Education and training will operate on two dimensions to support clinical governance. First, the education and training needed to generate the organisational awareness and commitment and support for systems and procedures. Second, the education and training needed to develop continuously the individual professionals level of knowledge and skills.

References

1   A First Class Service. Quality in the New NHS. *Health Services Circular*, 1998/113, at p. 33.
2   Ibid, at p. 33.
3   The future of SIFT, MADEL and NMET. Charles Easmon, February 1998.
4   A First Class Service. Quality in the New NHS. *Health Services Circular*, 1998/113, at p. 42.
5   The right team for the job. NHS Executive North Thames, October 1997 Glossary of terms, at pp. 54–64.
6   Ibid., Glossary of terms, at pp. 54–64.
7   Ibid., Glossary of terms, at pp. 54–64.
8   A First Class Service. Quality in the New NHS, at p. 42.
9   Ibid., at p. 35.
10 The New NHS. Modern. Dependable. CM3807, December 1997, at para. 6.10.
11 A First Class Service. Quality in the New NHS, at p. 44.
12 Ibid., at p. 45.
13 The New NHS. Modern. Dependable. CM3807, December 1997, at para. 7.15.

►12

The Role of the Medical Director

Jenny Simpson

'*The Medical Director is the guardian of clinical probity*' – Dr Alastair Scotland, October 1993, Medical Directors Group, the British Association of Medical Managers.

The complex and constantly evolving role of the Medical Director provides a fascinating perspective from which to view the development of clinical governance. The Medical Director in any NHS organisation is so closely involved in the development of clinical governance, it could perhaps be said that the principles of clinical governance more or less define the job of the Medical Director.

This chapter sets out to examine the role of the Medical Director – perhaps the most challenging in today's NHS. First, the context is set, by exploring the development of the role from the beginning, then moving on to discuss the nature of the job and the practical realities that face the Medical Director. The chapter concludes with a discussion of the skills and knowledge Medical Directors need to be able to do the job. The underlying thesis of the chapter is that in most organisations the Medical Director is the key player in clinical governance and that it is crucial for the long term health of the NHS that Medical Directors are educated and developed so that they can deliver these complex and challenging roles effectively and with confidence.

The early days

When trusts were first created, following the 1991 White Paper, *Working for patients*, the single uniting feature of the job was a singular lack of clarity. The White Paper had positioned the Medical Director as a statutory role, but the nature of the job was neither described nor defined. The ethos of the day was very much to let Trusts find their own way of developing the role and thus the job very much reflected the culture of the Trust itself.

Job descriptions and indeed contracts were either vague or entirely absent and for the first two years or so, each Medical Director's job was peculiar to the individual organisation. Medical Directors largely assumed that the role was representative, providing the medical staff view at the Trust board. At board meetings in the early days of Trusts, Medical Directors functioned very much as the former chairmen of medical staff committees and adopted much the same behaviour.

Early on, there were Medical Directors in post with no specific time allocated and no reward whatsoever. In reality, these individuals were regarded as mere figureheads with no real managerial influence to speak of. Over the first few months, many Medical Directors fell by the wayside, as it became clear that not only was the role extremely complex, but also that it demanded a great deal from the busy clinician.

As the months went by, it became very clear that the role had a number of different aspects. A striking phenomenon in the early days was the variation between Medical Director jobs – one Medical Director spent most of his management time finding beds for acute emergency admissions, whilst another was solely concerned with sorting out contracting arrangements with the then newly introduced fundholding general practitioners. With the passage of time, however, this new breed of professionals began to share their experiences somewhat and the role became more clearly defined, with discrete functions beginning to emerge.

Developing clear managerial relationships

Amongst the newly appointed Medical Directors, who on the whole were somewhat bewildered with their new positions, emerged a group of individuals who had a much clearer vision of what the role could and should be. By 1993–94, this group of doctors had taken on the role pro-actively and were determined to play a major role in the strategic direction of their Trusts. They set about developing clear managerial relationships, both with the Chief Executive and with Clinical Directors. This cadre of individuals which had been meeting under the auspices of the Medical Directors Group of the British Association of Medical Managers, transformed itself in April 1994 into the Association of Trust Medical Directors (ATMD) which sits within the BAMM organisation.

By the summer of 1996, the ATMD was in a position to produce a document entitled *The Roles and Responsibilities of the Medical Director*, based on an extensive survey of UK Medical Directors, which drew together the key common elements of the job. The circulation of this document also served to enlighten the NHS as to quite how broad and demanding the role of the Medical Director had become. On the other hand, it clearly also engendered some considerable anxiety in those Trusts where the Medical Director was not performing these duties or was trying to deliver the role with inadequate time, resources or skill.

Alongside the production of this document, Medical Directors had been developing their skills and knowledge at an impressive pace. Many had undertaken some form of management development, others had gained their skills by hard-earned experience. By the time *Roles and Responsibilities* was published, a major change had taken place. Medical Directors had begun to emerge as key strategic players in Trusts and it was generally agreed that the job simply could not be done on much less than a half-time commitment. Also, there was a distinct change in the type of person appointed to the post. Initially, the role seemed to be the domain of the pre-retirement consultant, the elder statesman, and the well-respected clinician getting towards the end of his or her career. These individuals were characterised by a determination not to rock the boat, to keep things on an even keel, and had largely acquired their positions by means of a tap on the shoulder from the Chief Executive, or as many described it, 'by not jumping back quickly enough when the chief executive was looking for volunteers'.

Broaden horizons

The newer breed of Medical Directors was most certainly younger. They also saw the opportunity of being a Medical Director as a strategic career step, as a chance to spread wings, broaden horizons and gain valuable experience. Many of this new breed had previously been involved in some form of management development, either through involvement in management projects or as a result of a personal commitment to understanding more about management. The new breed took the role very seriously, despite the fact that the drawbacks – the constant battle between managerial and clinical demands, the lack of any career progression for those taking on these roles and a lack of a reward system that would make the post attractive – were by now, only too clearly appreciated. These issues, which are still largely unresolved today, were fully recognised at this stage as being of critical, if the role were to attract the brightest and best clinicians.

That said, doctors were and remain, increasingly attracted to take on the job. Why should this be so? Given the ever increasing pressure and need to get the quality of clinical care right, the stress of balancing a clinical and a managerial career, with less than excellent rewards, why then should doctors take on these posts?

The answer lies in the satisfaction clinicians found in using the insight and skill gained over years and years of operational clinical practice, to improve services for patients. Many doctors have been utterly frustrated for years by working in a system that simply does not support the delivery of excellent health care to patients. This does not, on any account, reflect ill-will or idleness on anyone's part, but is the inevitable consequence of a structure in which those making the policy and managerial decisions do not have the insight and knowledge of those working at the coal face, on a day to day basis. Many Medical Directors have commented that though they may earn less and have much more in the way of hassle, they nevertheless prefer to work in a medical management role than in a pure clinical job. It is both intellectually demanding and constantly changing. The ever present need to develop a creative solution to complex and high level problems is challenging. However, many Medical Directors describe the sense of achievement when the apparently impossible is made to happen through smart thinking, effective persuasion and leadership, as being by far the most satisfying part of the job.

The last ten years has seen a major change in attitude on the part of medical professionals, from one in which management is a 'dirty word', its sole purpose being to thwart the effort of clinical professionals, to one in which every doctor has management as part of his or her job and the choice is whether to do that part well and with the appropriate knowledge and skill – or not. These changes, however, have not taken place at the same pace everywhere, nor has the environment of the NHS remained stable.

To-day's medical management environment

The last few years has seen major changes in the public's perception and indeed expectations of healthcare. In the past, the public had been happy to believe that 'doctor knows best' and was comfortable in accepting the doctor's superior knowledge base. The public was also largely unaware of major differences in either quality of, or access to, healthcare.

The rate of technological advance has been dramatic over the last decade and has radically altered what can be provided – and therefore what can be demanded and expected of the NHS. Alongside this, exposure on television documentaries of numerous service failures and the frank depiction of the medical world in television drama, 'soaps' and other media forms, have all contributed to a growing public awareness that doctors are indeed fallible human beings. Uncomfortable as this notion might be, the public has realised that health care standards in all parts of the country are by no means identical. The ease of access to resources of medical knowledge through the information superhighway has further empowered members of the public, who are not only becoming aware of the possibilities that healthcare could deliver but are also far less accepting of the concept of clinical freedom. All of this has led to a far less stable environment, a situation which has been further fuelled by a number of very public failures in the systems safeguarding the clinical probity of NHS organisations.

Most prominent in the public eye has been the Bristol heart surgery case in 1998, in which paediatric cardiac surgeons continued to operate despite clear evidence that they should no longer do so, given the mortality of the procedures in their hands. This case along with the failures of cancer screening services which hit the headlines throughout 1998 have served as a catalyst to the current thinking on clinical governance. Indeed, performance of clinical practitioners, along with a growing preoccupation with quality management systems and the added impetus of the failures have, between them, contributed in large measure to the quality management aspects of the Government's White Paper of December 1997, *The New NHS. Modern. Dependable.*

It is within this context that today's Medical Director works and lives. It is a fascinating and demanding role, which should not, on any account, be taken lightly. Above all, the role of Medical Director should not be undertaken by individuals without the appropriate aptitude, knowledge and skills. It is essential that the trust board ensures that the right individual with the right support, training, development and resources is appointed to this role which is so critical to the Trust's future health.

Clinical Governance and the Medical Director

In the new world of clinical governance, the Medical Director and his or her counterpart in nursing management are the key players in the Trust. The case study below outlines some of the issues involved.

● **Case study.** The issues

Dr Wellman, Medical Director at Heartwood Hospital was having a trying day. The chief cause of his concern was Andrew Thompson, the senior surgeon in the hospital. Although Andrew had no formal managerial role in the Trust he was nevertheless extremely influential as the 'elder statesman' surgeon. Gordon Wellman had become increasingly concerned about the infection rate from Andrew's team, particularly in his cholecystectomy patients. An audit had been undertaken 18 months previously and the audit team had felt that, as a whole, the surgical infection rates were high. The directorate team had drawn up a set of guidelines, and all the surgeons had agreed to change their practice. Now, 18 months on, although the infection rate across the directorate had improved, Andrew's rates were as high, if not higher than they were before.

Now Gordon had been acutely embarrassed by a conversation with Becky Morris, Nurse Manager in the Surgical Directorate. Becky had been concerned for some time about Mr Thompson's behaviour in theatre. He was rude and aggressive on many occasions and frequently late for lists. Furthermore, as she tartly observed, 'It's a waste of time drawing up guidelines – the good ones take them on board anyway, but Andrew won't listen to anyone but himself. He always does his own thing'.

Four miles across the city, at the Royal Hospital, Dr John Burton, Medical Director was frowning over the list of consultants applying for management training courses. He had masterminded the implementation of an appraisal system for all consultant staff two years previously. The initial first year had been extremely hard work, not only in terms of getting through the appraisal session with each of the 108 consultants, and the subsequent follow up personal development meetings, but also in terms of training the clinical directors in conducting the appraisals themselves. This year, however, the process had been somewhat less stressful with the Clinical Directors taking on much more of the load.

Dr Burton is keen to be as accommodating as possible to the consultants. However, each consultant has his or her clinical CME accredits to achieve, and time and resources are limited. The dilemma John Burton now faces is how to allocate the meagre management development budget fairly amongst the consultant staff, whilst at the same time ensuring that the skills and knowledge most needed by the Trust broadly matches those of the individuals. 'I have to say that what I think is needed and what they think they need are sometimes entirely different things' he mused, 'but I'm still really pleased that the colleagues are showing such enthusiasm.'

The management philosophy at the Royal, developed over the last five years between John Burton and Mark Winston, Chief Executive, was one of ensuring that effective systems are in place to monitor the quality of clinical practice. Thus, clinical audit, risk management, patient feedback, outcome measures and process improvement systems had been developed over the years in a structured programme, alongside an active approach to developing strong clinical leadership. These systems, however, are only ever as good as the individuals concerned, and the ability of these individuals to influence their clinical colleagues. The trust's executive team, having placed considerable emphasis on the systems development side over the last 5 years, is now fairly confident that quality failures will be picked up swiftly. The predominant emphasis now at the Royal is on developing individuals and encouraging them to adopt a more proactive approach – preventing disasters before they have a chance to happen.

The first duty of any Medical Director in delivering clinical governance must be to ensure that systems to pick up quality failures are in place. It is, however, all too easy to make the assumption that once the basic systems are in place, no more need be done, the box is checked and everyone can relax. Indeed it is crucial that Medical Directors fight against the inherent tendency to focus on systems, technology and committee structures as being the 'answer' to clinical governance.

It is fundamental that medical managers understand that the key to managing clinical performance, to achieving clinical governance, is mastering the art of influencing colleagues, peers with whom the individual has probably worked for many years and persuading them, at the very minimum, to improve their clinical performance, should it not be of an acceptable standard. At best, clinical governance is about creating an environment in which all clinical professionals are motivated and inspired to improve their clinical and professional performance, even though it is already of a high standard. Clearly the challenges that face the Medical Director vary greatly depending on the nature of the Trust and the type of management systems that are in place to monitor quality.

Developing the right culture

The basic management challenge, however, faces every Medical Director and is common to every Trust – that of developing the right culture to allow quality improvement to take place. The fact that has to be faced is that no one can change the individual's clinical practice, other than themselves. Information can be produced, mission statements can be issued, policies and guidelines can be circulated, persuasion, exhortation and peer pressure can be brought to bear – but unless the clinician has made a conscious decision to change or improve the way he or she performs, nothing will happen. Changing clinical behaviour is notoriously difficult. As the Nurse Manager in the case quite rightly observed, the 'good', conscientious clinicians, who indeed, are by far in the majority, are keen to improve their practice anyway – after all, no clinician sets off to do the job poorly in the first place. However, there is a small number of doctors who are simply unwilling to change their practice and indeed do not see any need so to do.

Clinical governance aims to develop and enhance clinical practice amongst the good, whilst simultaneously providing a set of systems to ensure that poor practice is identified, the lessons learnt implemented into clinical practice and the effect of these lessons monitored.

The two Trusts described in the case have very different approaches and have very different perspectives on the introduction of clinical governance. However, the huge difference between the organisations is only really appreciated by the small number of clinical staff who hold sessions in both Trusts.

● **Case study.** Three months later

Back at Heartwood hospital, things are not going at all well. Andrew Thompson lost his temper with a senior theatre nurse last week, swore at her and was both threatening and abusive to her. The scene was witnessed by Dr Malcolm Neil, a newly appointed Consultant Anaesthetist. Dr Neil works mainly at the Royal but also covers two lists each week at Heartwood and had recently taken on Andrew Thompson's list. Dr Neil is hoping to take over as clinical director of anaesthesia at the Royal and has a keen interest in quality management models.

'I am just appalled by this man's behaviour,' he mused to himself 'but what is the right thing to do? The management lot at Heartwood don't seem to be interested and yet this man is going to do some real damage before too long – if he's not already done so? We have ways of picking all this up at the Royal, but nothing here at Heartwood so I'm now left with the question of whether I should report him. If I do, it's not going to win me any friends – but if I don't, maybe *I'm* in the wrong. I'm sure the latest guidance from the GMC makes that clear.' Finally Dr Neil decides to have an informal chat with John Burton at the Royal who whilst busy, as always, is happy to spend half an hour chewing over the matter.

Meanwhile at Heartwood, Gordon Wellman had just received a formal complaint about Andrew Thompson from Becky Morris. He was at his desk, considering the next steps when the telephone rang. 'The Chairman and I wondered if you could pop over for a few minutes?' the Trust's chief executive Paul Johnson said, 'We've got some pretty serious complaints we need to discuss with you.' Dr Wellman made his way over to the Executive Offices with a heavy heart.

Over at the Royal, Dr Neil was feeling somewhat more optimistic. He had had the chance to talk things through with John Burton and had decided to confront both Gordon Wellman and Paul Johnson at Heartwood the next day.

The nuts and bolts of clinical governance must be in place at directorate or service level. The Medical Director cannot and should not personally oversee every consultant or process. With the development of clinical governance, the Medical Director's role becomes quite clear. As the guardian of clinical probity, the Medical Director must be confident that effective systems and effective clinical leadership are in place for each and every clinical service within the Trust. That said, the Medical Director must also know how to deal effectively, appropriately and skilfully with the clinician whose performance is falling below the expected standard.

This is often a complex business, with multiple aspects. The colleague may be ill, may be stressed, may be behaving in an unacceptable manner or may be incompetent. However, most problems with colleagues do not present with a single convenient label on them. Most are multifaceted, with information presenting from every direction and sporadically. The Medical Director must constantly be on the alert for patterns of unusual behavior amongst clinical colleagues. The Medical Director must be close enough to the action to know when things are going wrong and to be closely connected to the internal, informal networks of the Trust. At the same time, however, he or she must also stand back sufficiently to view the organisation as a whole and set the issues within the right context.

It is the Medical Director's responsibility to make sure that the culture and environment is one in which poor performance and clinical risk are managed with skill and sensitivity. Consultants and particularly clinical directors must be made fully aware of how much of the monitoring and indeed investigation of effective performance should be undertaken and at what stage the matter should be reported to the Medical Director. There must, of course, be a full and open relationship between the Medical Director, Clinical Director and consultant colleagues. Without this, the Medical Director can not hope to be successful in clinical governance.

Develop the informal network

Consider the Trusts outlined in the case. At the Royal, considerable effort has been put into developing a system. The philosophy of the Trust is clearly articulated, at every step of the management process. The process, which provides a useful vehicle for discussing performance and the needs for further professional development, also provides a mechanism for managing staff morale and health. An important by-product, however, is the opportunity the process provides to develop the informal network, to gain the soft information of who is doing what – and which areas of the Trust the Medical Director might wish to focus on most clearly. The appraisal process makes staff feel valued. It is unfortunate to note that an approach like this remains somewhat unusual in today's NHS. As one consultant remarked, rather sadly, 'this is the first time anyone has ever asked or cared about what I do next'.

In contrast, at Heartwood, each and every problem in the service will come as an unpleasant surprise, simply because the ethos of proactively seeking out the problems is not there and Gordon Wellman does not have the 'inside knowledge' he needs to be effective. The Trust management is therefore set on the back foot and is constantly reacting to issues that could and should have been prevented.

There are many and varied calls upon the Medical Director's time. As most Medical Directors are still working clinically, time is indeed under pressure. However, of all the many things a Medical Director must do, this determination to create the right culture and the right networks is top priority. Without it, the role as a Medical Director is totally reactive and as such is not really manageable. At the Royal, John Burton has created a culture which will support him in his job, by means of an appraisal system. There are in fact many other ways and other systems that can be used as a mechanism to change the culture of an organisation and the true art is identifying the mechanism most likely to bring about change, given the nature of the Trust.

● **Case study.** The next day

Malcolm Neil arrived early for his list at Heartwood hospital. He had arranged to have a word with Gordon Wellman and Paul Johnson before he went to theatre, although now he was beginning to question the wisdom of his actions. His confidence of the previous evening had evaporated on his arrival at Heartwood, and now he desperately wished he had kept quiet. As he began to explain his concerns to the Medical Director and Chief Executive he sensed that Gordon Wellman was already somewhat stressed and irritated at his remarks. Paul Johnson on the other hand listened calmly and encouraged Malcolm to expand on his anxieties about Andrew Thompson's performance. 'It's no use avoiding the issue any more. Something's just got to be done!' Gordon Wellman was almost shouting, 'Why is this sort of thing always happening here? Can't we have some sort of quality policy in this place to stop all this nonsense?' Malcolm Neil was not terribly sure what to say about all this but began anyway to describe some of the processes in place at the Royal. Again Paul Johnson listened carefully and Malcolm left for his list feeling that at least no harm had been done.

Two days later John Burton at the Royal was slightly surprised to hear from Paul Johnson at Heartwood. Paul had spoken to Mark Winston and had asked if both Chief Executives and Medical Directors could get together one evening for a drink to explore the possibility of sharing the Royal's approach to performance management with colleagues at Heartwood.

It is not easy to be a Medical Director. In many ways the introduction of clinical governance has clarified many of the issues, but at the same time has given the role considerable breadth and complexity, along with accountability for the fundamental in healthcare – the quality of clinical practice. It is essential that Medical Directors do the job well – a poorly performing Medical Director does no-one any service and can cause considerable damage.

So what makes a good Medical Director?

▶ First and foremost must come judgement. Just as in the clinical world, the facts and figures may be there, the why's and wherefore's evident. The real skill, however, lies in the Medical Director's judgement, timing, sensitivity and knowledge of how both the individuals and the organisation itself will react – and his or her ability to use this skill to make things happen.

▶ Second there is a menu of skills without which the Medical Director simply cannot survive. In terms of the clinical governance agenda, these must include risk and crisis management – and dealing with the poorly performing colleagues. Medical Directors must also know enough about the systems that should be in place to spot when they are not functioning properly. Medical Directors must above all know when the limits of their own knowledge have been reached – and they must certainly not be too proud to ask for help when they know they are in trouble.

▶ Finally – and perhaps this should come first, Medical Directors should know how to communicate effectively – not only with patients but also with colleagues, at board level, with the public, with the other clinical disciplines and with the media. All the knowledge and skill is useless if the ideas are not communicated effectively. If the key to buying a new business property is location, location, location, then the key to effective Medical Directoring must be communicate, communicate, communicate.

This may all seem a daunting prospect – and yet the real opportunity afforded by clinical governance must not be ignored by Medical Directors. Clinical governance provides not only a framework for the task of the Medical Director, but also provides the legitimacy and the power to demand demonstrable standards of quality in clinical care. For years clinicians – even those in medical management positions – have struggled with improving service quality, without the benefit of a nationally driven framework. Clinical governance provides that framework. It is now time for clinicians and medical managers in particular to demonstrate their determination to make clinical governance a reality and to make a real difference to the quality of care the NHS provides.

● Case study. Clinical governance and the Medical Director

▶ Clinical governance happens at directorate or service level – the Medical Director's job is to create the right environment to liberate and empower Clinical Directors to deliver clinical governance, through leadership and management systems.

▶ The Medical Director, along with management and clinical colleagues, should regard the development of a proactive, energetic approach to managing the quality of clinical performance as his or her topmost priority.

▶ The Medical Director must take every step to ensure that each clinical service or specialty
    (a) has effective and efficient clinical leadership
    (b) has high quality management and information systems.

▶ The Medical Director must be able to demonstrate with confidence that, for each service or specialty, the quality of clinical care is monitored, and when lacking that lessons are learnt and implemented.

▶ The Medical Director must develop robust informal networks with the Clinical Directors, other clinicians and managers which will allow a detailed knowledge and 'feel' for the organisation whilst simultaneously keeping an organisation–wide perspective.

▶ Communication, time management, investigation and influencing skills are key requirements.

References

Roles and Responsibilities of the Medical Director, published by the Association of Trust Medical Directors, ISBN 1 900120 02X.

The New NHS. Modern. Dependable, Cmd 3807, published December 1997 by the Department of Health.

▶13

Information, Data Quality and Clinical Governance

Dipak Kalra, David Patterson and David Ingram

Introduction

The White Paper, *The new NHS. Modern. Dependable*, sets the context for the clinical governance initiative. 'Every patient who is treated in the NHS wants to know that he or she can rely on receiving high-quality care when needed. Every part of the NHS, and everyone, who works in it, should take responsibility for working to improve quality'.[1] Implementation of the White Paper will bring everyone within the Service, as well as patients and their carers, into new working relationships and accountability. Clinical governance is a catalyst for the development of a unifying culture, which recognises and upholds the maintenance and improvement of quality as the heart of the service to patients.

Achieving the goals of clinical governance will crucially depend upon the development of new roles and skills within clinical practice and new information systems to guide and support them. There is no failure-proof 'blue print' to guide such developments – they will evolve through experience and this will take time.

The main thrust of the information strategy, Information for Health,[2] is to shift the focus of quality within healthcare organisations, away from administrative efficiency and towards support of clinicians' work. The White Paper aims to achieve improvement in the health outcomes of individual patients and in their experience of care delivery. This will require the efficient application of evidence-based clinical interventions in multi-professional teams, coordinated within many institutional and domestic settings. There will be growing opportunities for patients to be more directly involved in their own care, through eduction, support in the home and the self-reporting of personal health status and needs.

The key to success lies in harnessing and developing the skills and experience of clinicians working in healthcare teams. The clinical requirements, for which information technology will increasingly be utilised, are in the areas of:

▶ developing an integrated knowledge environment that delivers evidence about best practice, clinical guidelines and educational materials directly to the clinical 'coal face'

▶ improving multi-professional partnerships and clinical decision-making through ethically and legally acceptable access to patient record information and enhanced communication systems

▶ promoting systematic clinical practice, for example through data templates, clinical protocols and integrated care pathways, embedded within patient records providing patients with relevant education and support to enable good practice in their own self-management

 enhancing clinical performance by collecting feedback from patients on the various aspects of their care

stimulating a culture of evidence-based practice by linking results from clinical audit with professional educational programmes and resources.

Despite considerable progress made, the development of an integrated information system, which can link together clinical knowledge, interventions and records, securely, rigorously, and cost-effectively, and at the coal face of practice, remains a huge challenge. Achieving the transition from the systems of today to those required to meet the clinical governance vision of tomorrow is an extremely complex set of linked clinical, technical and managerial challenges.

This chapter primarily addresses clinical and informatics challenges faced in delivering an information systems environment to support clinical governance. Inevitably, this involves some consideration of technical issues, since these constrain feasible solutions.

Medicine and information technology

Zimmerli described information technology as '... the one and only "horizontal technology", a technology that pervades each and every part of social life and all the other technologies as well'.[3] Medical science might lay claim to being a 'horizontal science', on similar grounds. The marriage of the two is a uniquely rich encounter!

The broad range of applications of information technology is summarised in a definition of the field of informatics as '... the rational scientific treatment, notably by computer, needed to support knowledge and communications in technical, economic and social domains'.[4] Thirty years ago, the interdisciplinary field linking medicine and information technology was termed 'medical computing', a rather limited, technical connotation of how the two might interact.

With the growth of artificial intelligence research in the next decade, medicine laid claim to a field of 'medical informatics', defined as '... the rapidly developing scientific field that deals with resources, devices, and formalised methods for optimising the storage, retrieval, and management of biomedical information for problem solving and decision making'.[5] This recognised the emerging role of the computer as an essential component of new methods and tools of medical practice. Not to be out-done, disciplines of nursing and dental informatics appeared alongside!

The past decade has been characterised, worldwide, by growing awareness of the processes of healthcare delivery in achieving clinical effectiveness. Much greater emphasis on healthcare management, not simply healthcare administration, as had hitherto prevailed, and on the patient's perspective, as the recipient or customer for the service, led to crystallisation of a discipline of 'health informatics'. This '... examines the organisational, professional and technical issues involved in the use of information systems to support patient-centred healthcare delivery. It includes activities like clinical decision making, efficient information management, knowledge acquisition and dissemination, and informed patient participation'.[6]

Highest achievable quality

The task of defining, building and supporting the information infrastructures required to enable the cost-effective delivery of healthcare services, of the highest achievable quality, is inevitably very complex. Reasons for the fragmented and often chaotic progress made have been:

▶ rapid scientific and technological advance – and related problems of obsolescence

▶ diverse interests and expectations of stakeholders

▶ strong interactions between information technology and approaches to clinical practice and the delivery of healthcare

▶ weak conceptual framework and standards

▶ requirements and cost/benefits of innovations proving difficult to evaluate

▶ difficult and rather discouraging environment for business.

Progress in marrying the clear potential of information technology to the evolving needs of patients, clinicians and managers has also been a difficult human challenge, due to:

▶ problems of understanding, roles and participation

▶ concurrent professional, service and organisational change

▶ adverse public reactions to costly and wasteful innovations yielding low perceived benefits

▶ feelings that there were many fine words and concepts, but few practical exemplars.

It is, therefore, not too surprising that the exceptionally fast-moving field of health informatics has a history characterised to an unhappy extent by costly and hurried innovation, limited and often disorganised application and rapid obsolescence. It has also proved very difficult to develop an adequate conceptual and strategic grasp of the field to guide investment. That said, and as the following sections seek to illustrate, significant progress has been achieved in understanding the requirements of clinical information management. The capability of information technology to satisfy these emerging requirements of real clinical practice has evolved hugely.

There is, however, much still to be learned about the effective deployment of information technology in support of healthcare. In the meantime, Health Services must cope with the pressing immediate needs of the patients and populations they serve. New clinical information management skills will be fundamental to coping with the changing culture of healthcare implied by clinical governance, where patients' perspectives and the quality of clinical outcomes achieved are made explicit driving forces within the service.

Effectiveness of clinical services

The White Paper builds on a trend of increasing emphasis on scientific method to justify the effectiveness of clinical services. It proposes wider public and multi-professional involvement, for example through primary care groups, in the setting of priorities and in the delivery of programmes for health improvement of the population. Marrying informatics to the needs of these groups is a major challenge. It is arguable, though, that the new NHS vision cannot be realised without considerable progress in this area.

The objective to provide cost-effective and timely clinical treatments and services, based on scientific foundations of proven efficacy and prioritised to meet health needs for diverse populations, are easily stated but difficult to conceptualise, communicate and deliver. They have to bridge from the local to national and international perspectives, since health issues now, more than ever, link the world together at all times and in all places.

Healthcare information systems must enable coherent and reliable access to:

▶ scientific knowledge, which provides the foundations of clinical practice

▶ clinical standards for intervention protocols and decision support

▶ clinical records

▶ tools for audit of the cost and quality of care delivered, from both patient and professional perspectives

▶ educational resources – both to support patient self-care and to enable continuing education for professionals.

The integration of different kinds of information required to support performance of an individual clinical intervention is illustrated in Figure 13.1.

This information must be coherent with many other areas of knowledge about people, institutions and services, within and beyond healthcare, for example Patients' Support Groups, Prisons and Social Services. Such diverse groupings may have very different needs and perspectives on healthcare information and its management. Development, dissemination and maintenance of high quality clinical and technical standards for information, in the public domain, are essential for an orderly approach to the management of this diversity. They are vital for a single institution and locality as much as they are nationally and internationally.

International differences in clinical practice are perhaps lesser obstacles to progress than protective self-interest and tradition within countries and professions. Achieving useful steps forward in the quality of information management, while retaining the richness of this diversity, is a painstaking process but an important and achievable goal.

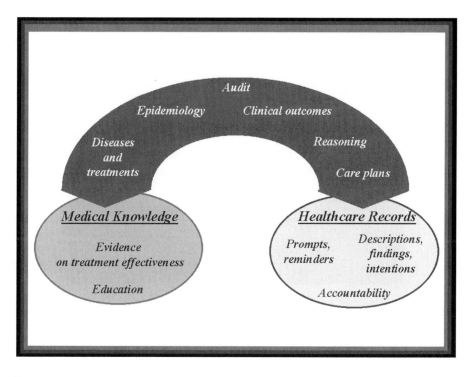

Fig. 13.1.   The domains of information relevant to a clinical intervention.

Information requirements in a changing health service

The management of healthcare has traditionally implied an information flow through the service as depicted within Figure 13.2. This is rather a top-down perspective on the management of information. Data is collected and information flows to serve a contractual model of healthcare delivery and finance. Quality and resource trade-offs determining services provided are adjudicated at the higher levels.

Figure 13.3, from an article by Smith,[7] suggests that traditional models of healthcare services have been associated with inefficient and inequitable healthcare, where expensive specialised interventions are favoured, as characterised by the upper triangle. At the same time, some more useful measures, to provide support for patients and families at home, are under-resourced. It suggests that information technology may enable a new concept of service as illustrated in the lower triangle, aiming to correct this balance by creating a more patient and information-centred view of healthcare. Quality measures would focus more on individual patient's needs and experiences of care they received. Services would be encouraged which

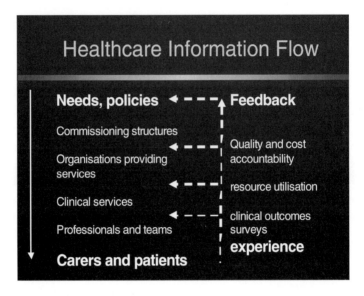

Fig. 13.2. A top-down view of healthcare information.

met these needs through involving the patient fully in their individual self-management and which were delivered as near to the patient's home and community as possible. This would open many new choices for patients, with resources and professional roles structured to support these choices. Such a model,

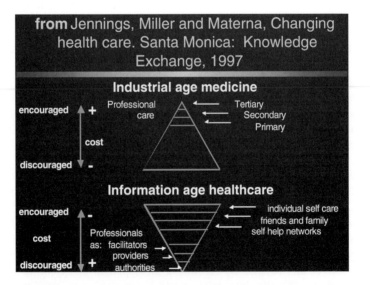

Fig. 13.3. Evolution from the traditional hospital-centred view towards a patient-centred and distributed view of healthcare services, supported by information technology.

depends on the capacity of information technology to support people, communications and workflow in the highly distributed teams and interventions which are implied.

We started this chapter with the observation that clinical governance is a catalyst for change. Much of the White Paper describes policies for moving from a Figure 13.2 towards a Figure 13.3 concept of healthcare. Here, quality as well as cost and ethico-legal requirements lie at the heart of the regulation of service delivery. Human and financial resource management, especially in education, is the most important driving force of this change. The information systems required will change radically as patients become more involved in the delivery and support of their care.

Future trends

Whatever these future trends, much else is already changing at the coalface of clinical interventions. Healthcare professionals need to document increasing volumes of information, as patients receive increasingly complex care, involving a range of data-intensive examinations, investigations and treatments. The majority of clinical detail in records and in communications is still on paper.[8] To cope with this complexity, there is a movement from a highly narrative to a more structured style of record keeping. This is taking place at a different pace in different disciplines. It is likely that narratives will always have a place to document a patient's story or to capture the more discursive elements of a patient's management.[9]

Clinicians need to keep more detailed records to demonstrate their competence[10] in case of future litigation, which is increasing in frequency each year, and in order to justify their use of healthcare resources. They also need to share healthcare information with a wider range of professional colleagues on multiple sites. The care of any one patient can require a healthcare professional to review the information held in several distributed clinical systems in a consistent manner.[11]

Clinicians and managers require high quality tools to analyse the data within patient records[12] in order to:

▶ observe trends and patterns in the health of a patient

▶ enable the use of clinical guidelines and decision support systems as part of evidence-based practice

▶ perform clinical audit

▶ inform management and commissioning decisions

▶ support epidemiology, research and teaching activities.

Patients can acquire considerable expertise in managing their own health if they are given useful and appropriate material with which to educate themselves.[13,14] The ability to tailor such educational materials to individual needs, and to make them available at times and in locations suitable to each patient are important for the success of modern shared care. Feedback to patients and to clinicians is also vital if such information is to result in lasting behaviour changes.

Health services, internationally, are grappling with the evolution from paper-based to electronic healthcare record systems. There are many perceived benefits of using computers to capture, organise and view healthcare record data. Duplicate data entry can be avoided if information is captured, maintained and communicated securely and consistently, in line with clinical needs. The same information can be displayed and viewed in a variety of ways, for example by problem or episode or through summaries, as well as in the traditional chronological order. Standard datasets and templates to assist in their capture and communication can be defined and adapted as practice evolves. The patient record may be accessed from any terminal on a network (even by multiple users simultaneously), and communicated electronically to support seamless shared care. Routine data analyses and the records systems which enable and support shared care protocols can also be implemented.

Present day clinical information systems in hospitals and in general practice are not adequate for the challenges of delivering effective and evidence-based healthcare, in which teams of clinicians on different sites are working in partnership and collaboratively with patients.[15] The experience of many healthcare professionals (especially in hospitals) is that the clinical computer systems available to them are too slow or cumbersome for use in a realistic consultation time.[16] The diversity and complexity of clinical data cannot be captured fully and faithfully on most contemporary systems.[17,18] Duplication of data entry often still occurs because the existing paper folders are usually retained in addition to newly computerised record systems.[19]

It has been estimated that 15% of the resources of an acute hospital are spent in gathering and processing information, accounting for up to 25% of doctor and nurse time.[20] So there is clearly much scope for improving the efficiency of clinical information management. Electronic and paper healthcare records are held in islands of information in independent information systems, each with its own technical characteristics and view of the healthcare domain. The available evidence on good clinical practice, existing as publications and guidelines, is often too generalised to be applied to individual patient groups, and is isolated from the relevant known facts about any particular patient's medical and social background.[21] This evidence is difficult to retrieve at the time and in the location where needed. For these kinds of reasons, clinical audit has proved difficult to integrate into daily practice without specific facilitation.[22] It is extremely difficult to deliver optimum care when these practical clinical requirements are not satisfied.

Components of evidence-based information systems for healthcare

Clinicians and patients need high-quality information systems to connect an individual person or healthcare record to a repository of the knowledge that is relevant to the care provided. A number of key information system components are required in order to build an information systems environment that can meet the requirements of an evidence-based and patient-focused healthcare service (Fig. 13.4).

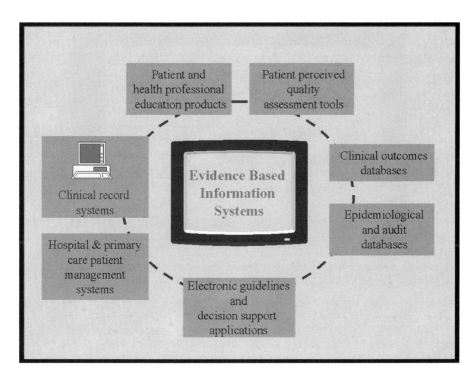

Fig. 13.4. The computer system components required to support evidence-based and outcomes-oriented clinical practice.

A comprehensive electronic healthcare record (EHCR) that can be used to capture all of the necessary healthcare information traditionally held in paper records, including:

▶ free-text

▶ units of measurement, normal ranges and accuracy

▶ radiological images and bio-signals

▶ templates and standard data sets

▶ term set entries, with qualifiers, synonyms and abbreviations

▶ charts, tables, drawing and diagrams

▶ drug prescriptions, standard letters and reports, patient summaries.

When migrating to electronic healthcare records, it is important to acknowledge the tremendous richness of clinical and contextual information that can be expressed very elegantly on paper (see Fig. 13.5). EHCR systems need to offer a flexible framework

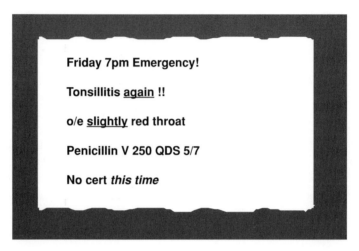

Fig. 13.5. An example of a narrative record entry, showing the subtle doctor-patient interactions that can be expressed within a few lines of text.

for recording the consultation process, and accommodate the individuality of the clinician as well as the patient.

Clinical practice requires a rich and varied vocabulary to express the diversity and complexity of each patient encounter. An EHCR system must be underpinned by a common terminology to express clinical content, that can accommodate such freedom of expression, whilst supporting the need for structured and semi-structured interpretation of each entry.

The way in which individual clinical statements are hierarchically nested within a record confers an important context for their interpretation. A comprehensive EHCR system must enable statements to be grouped together under headings and sub-headings in a clinically meaningful way. Aspects of certainty, severity and the absence of findings must be capable of rigorous and unambiguous representation. For example, a patient with only a family history of diabetes or in whom diabetes has been excluded must not erroneously be retrieved in a database search for diabetic patients.

Electronic healthcare records must be medico-legally acceptable, for example as legal evidence, with a rigorous audit trail of authorship and amendments. They must be implemented within a formal security and access framework that ensures only the appropriate persons connected with the care of the patient can retrieve and edit their record.

In a teaching setting, it must be possible for medical, nursing and other healthcare students to have access to and to contribute to healthcare records, such that their student status is explicit. The patient (and possibly their families) must themselves be valid authors of record entries to allow them to contribute their own impressions of health status and needs.

EHCR systems must be implemented within a secure communications infrastructure that allows for the seamless integration of existing (legacy) computer systems whilst these remain in use, and for the ongoing inclusion of new-generation systems. Healthcare information must be transferred between sites in a secure manner and comply with both NHS[23] and European[24,25,26] directives.

A set of standard clinical protocols that can be adapted and customised for use in individual patients or for specific patient groups. These protocols must be capable of drawing on information already contained within a patient's record, without requiring duplicate data entry. They must be capable of being transferred along with a patient's record so that the same protocol can be followed with the patient at different locations. Some aspects of protocols will be applicable to patient self-management, such as advice on the manipulation of insulin doses in relation to the home monitoring of blood glucose in a diabetic patient.

An integrated medical knowledge environment incorporating on-line databases (such as Medline, drugs databases, clinical effectiveness literature and electronic guidelines of best practice). These might be accessed as look-up options directly from screens within a clinical system and might need to be incorporated, as pointers within a healthcare record, to show justification of clinical decisions and actions taken. The use of directed Internet-based resources for patients and healthcare professionals have been documented in several settings, for example.[27]

A multi-media education environment to provide simple guidance or detailed background information, for professionals and for patients. This might be accessed directly through menus and keyword searches and used as part of organised dedicated educational sessions, or linked through pointers, from an individual patient's record. Such materials will progressively incorporate assessments of skills and knowledge acquired, to provide a means for health professional accreditation.

A rich set of client software tools, for example to present the large volumes of accumulated information in a user-friendly manner, to counter the dangers of information overload, and to allow for views of trends and patterns in the progress of individual patients and across sub-populations.

The progressive incorporation of evaluation tools, such as questionnaires and standard queries on the underlying clinical databases, to provide feedback on the structure, process and outcome of healthcare provision.

The foregoing is not intended as a comprehensive list of possible components. It is designed to give a feel for the way in which clinical requirements must be met in building towards an information environment which supports the objectives of clinical governance. Many other components will be required to integrate the whole information environment, especially to ensure secure and accountable data entry, retrieval and communication.

Examples of relevant development projects in Europe

The NHS Information Management Group has developed a wide range of projects over many years in building towards an electronic communications infrastructure for the NHS. Amongst the most notable tasks has been the development of a set of standard messages to enable the transfer of managerial and clinical information between purchasers and providers[28] over the new NHS network. The expansion of the initial set of Read codes, through the Clinical Terms Project, aims to provide a 'language for healthcare' for new generations of clinical systems.[29] The Electronic Patient Record Project has highlighted many of the difficulties which must be overcome if the hospital medical record is to be fully computerised.[30] The new NHS Information Strategy[2] defines a formal and funded commitment to the integration of patient records within hospitals (Electronic Patient Records) and across the wider NHS (Electronic Healthcare Records).

The Health Telematics Research and Development programme of the European Union has recognised many of these health informatics challenges and sought to address them on a larger scale through a set of multi-national projects over the past decade.[31,32] The main projects on electronic healthcare have included the Good European Health Record (GEHR) and Synapses projects.

The Good European Health Record (GEHR) project was established to develop a common health record architecture, published in the public domain, for Europe.[33] The project consortium comprised 21 organisations in seven EU countries and included clinicians from different professions and disciplines, computer scientists in commercial and academic institutions, and multi-national industrial partners. The project explored the clinical requirements for the wide-scale adoption of Electronic Healthcare Records (EHCRs) instead of paper records within primary and secondary care and across specialities. It also developed and evaluated prototypes based on a proposed standard architecture in these settings.

Clinical and technical requirements

Doctors, nurses and other allied professionals from across Europe were involved in deriving a set of clinical and technical requirements covering:

▶ comprehensive recording of healthcare data for a full range of disciplines in primary and secondary care[34]

▶ portability of healthcare records between hardware platforms, operating systems and applications[35]

▶ transfer of healthcare records via telecommunications networks or smart cards[36]

▶ ethical, medico-legal and security issues which arise when EHCRs are the sole medium for capturing, storing and communicating patient-related information[37]

▶ education, at undergraduate and postgraduate level, to enable the clinical workforce to utilise these new technologies.[38]

The results of the project strongly emphasised the priority of the rights of the individual patient when handling personal healthcare data within electronic records. It recognised, nonetheless, the requirement that, at times, clinicians will wish to review trends or activities in a consistent manner across sets of patients, Figure 13.6.

The most important publication from the GEHR project was a rigorous formal model of health record architecture, based on the specific clinical requirements referenced above. Computer system developers are building on this work. The GEHR requirements have contributed to subsequent European standards work in the field,[39] and new EU telematics projects, such as Synapses have built on these foundations.

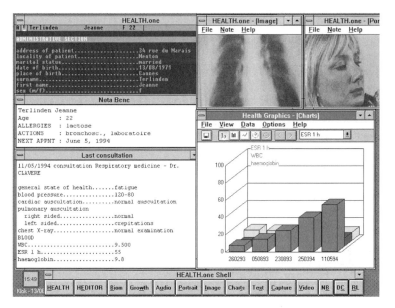

Fig. 13.6. Example screen from Health One (Health Data Management Partners, Brussels) developed during the GEHR project.

Research in the EU Synapses project has addressed the harmonisation of diverse healthcare record systems to enable clinicians to access information from any institution with electronic records about their patients.[40] The Synapses approach ensures that the original meaning of an entry is preserved when it is transferred to or viewed through another healthcare system.[41]

Preservation of clinical meaning

The preservation of clinical meaning within the EHCR hinges on use of shared or compatible terminologies for capturing clinical statements. The EU GALEN project has pioneered work in the formal representation of clinical concept models, and their cross-mapping to classification systems such as ICD and Read.[42] Further work is being undertaken in the UK, under the auspices of the NHS, to explore the extent to which clinical meaning and other kinds of context[43] can be represented reliably through record headings.[44] This work is informing the work of European Project teams developing proposals for new Council for European Normalisation (CEN) standards for term lists for EHCR communications.[45]

Electronic healthcare communications must take place within an appropriate professional and technical security framework. The EU Projects SEISMED[46,47] and ISHTAR[48] have investigated the clinical and legislative requirements and the available products across Europe. This work has informed drafting of the EU Data Protection Directive and related national legislation on patient-related data.[23,24]

Current EU projects, such as SynEx[49] and Prompt[50] are developing methods for integrating clinical protocols and medical knowledge environments with patient records systems.

As discussed, much of the work and experience gained in these illustrative projects has informed progress on standards through CEN and now in the International Standards Organisation. A four-part EHCR draft standard will be published during 1999.[51] The Project teams and titles are shown in Table 13.1.

Table 13.1.   Project Teams developing the new 4-part CEN standard on EHCR Communication.

PT-26	Part 1: Extended Architecture and Domain Model for the Electronic Healthcare Record
PT-27	Part 2: Domain Termlist
PT-28	Part 3: Distribution Rules
PT-29	Part 4: Messages for Exchange of Information

Experience of working to improve the quality of information to support patient care

Using common data sets

In order to support consistent shared care and allow clinical audit to take place across a range of clinical settings, the data collected must represent a consensus on what should be carried out and recorded in different situations. There are several reasons why it may be of benefit to agree on a common data-set to record the clinical content of, for example, the progress review of a chronic condition:

 The data set may act as a checklist to encourage consistent care of a high quality.

 The common use of identically structured records may facilitate shared care between hospitals, general practices and community health teams; this might also help with communications when patients move and change their GP or hospital.

 Common paper and computerised record structures can improve the scope for the subsequent analysis of recorded data, and enable easier collaborative (multi-site) audit.

▶ A standard approach to specific clinical conditions should enable the development of common educational materials for healthcare professionals, for patients and carers, and for students.

However, there are several practical issues to be addressed before a common data-set can be agreed and implemented across a large organisation or health district. Some of these are listed in Table 13.2.

Table 13.2. Challenges to be addressed before defining a standard clinical data-set.

Practical challenges to be addressed before defining a clinical data set
What is a realistic clinical review checklist (e.g. for a diabetes annual check)?
What is the best way for the checklist data to be recorded (in both paper and computerised records)?
How should a recent clinical review be communicated (on paper or via the computer)?
How can clinical care be best and most easily audited?
How can patients and their carers become involved (e.g. in providing their experience about clinical outcomes)?
Will extra resources be required to implement this programme across the organisation/district?
What benefits should be demonstrated in order to justify investment?

Standardised templates, proformas and summary sheets have increasingly been adopted across all sectors of healthcare. Many different kinds of data-sets may be used by healthcare professionals, including:

▶ forms and templates to collect or analyse patient information

▶ structured reports and referrals, including those reports required by Institutions or the Health Service about individual patients

▶ term sets, pick-lists (Fig. 13.7) and screen layouts incorporated within clinical applications

▶ data to be analysed across patient populations for clinical audit or departmental reporting requirements

▶ messages used in communication, e.g. with a local healthcare purchasing authority

▶ local research or teaching databases for which patient information is collected and analysed.

The design of forms, for paper or computer use, should facilitate rapid and structured data entry catering for the majority of possible responses. This might include the use of anatomical diagrams, tick-boxes, pick-lists and preferred terms from a term-set. However, it is important to incorporate some flexibility to allow for unique individual findings and for the recording of additional personal details. When this flexibility is

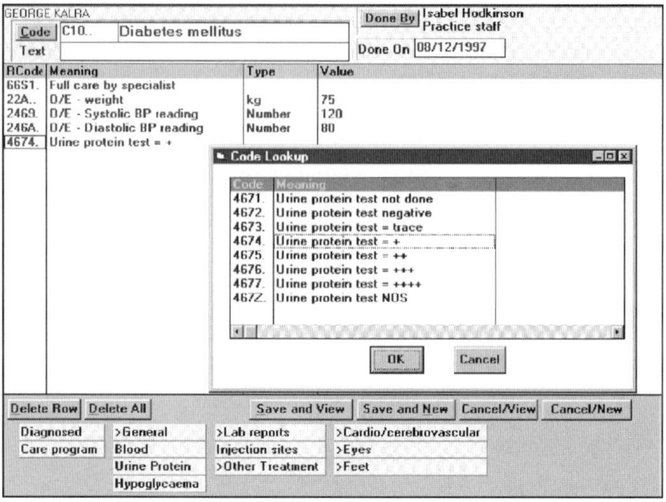

Fig. 13.7. Example computer screen showing pick-lists during data entry within a Diabetes Protocol (GP-CARE: CHIME, University College London).

absent, forms tend not to be completed and professionals need to return to a more traditional narrative recording style.

The process of developing each common data-set must not be taken as a goal in itself, but should form part of a total quality strategy for the service to a particular patient group.

Relating guidelines to patient records

Clinical guidelines are systematically developed statements designed to assist practitioners to decide about appropriate healthcare in specific clinical circumstances.[52] Most hospitals and general practices are developing a range of templates or protocols of care which embody published evidence on clinical effectiveness expressed in the form of algorithmic guidelines. Historically, it has proved difficult to integrate guidelines within everyday clinical practice and to ensure that they remain an effective tool when used during patient consultations.[53] Patient encounters are usually hurried, with many agendas to meet within severe time pressures. This makes it a difficult setting in which to think strategically, to practise effectively or to deliver educational messages. Clinical guidelines are renowned for lying on shelves, unread and untouched.

The presentation of useful patient-specific reminders, provided by clinical systems during consultations, seems to improve adherence to guidelines.[54] A paper-based, integrated record and guideline, known as the Integrated Care Pathway (ICP) has been adopted in a number of hospitals. Figure 13.8 shows a section from an ICP for the management of a fractured neck of femur at the Whittington Hospital in North London. The complete ICP comprises over 50 templates that combine guidance notes and spaces for capturing the record of care given, spanning a patient's admission,

---

Assess Pain - F & G Grade A&E Nursing Staff

a) Record Pain Score from diagram below - Pain Score ....score

b) Give Pain Relief as per standing order below

Pain Measurement	Drug	Dose	Route
1-5	Co-dydramol	2 tabs	Orally
5-10	Pethidine	50 mgs	Intra-muscular
Nausea from Pethidine	Prochlorperazine(Stemetil)	12.5 mgs	Intra-muscular

Medication & Dose...Time Given.........................

Complete R_x (Treatment Chart) ☐ ....initials

Assess Pressure Area Risk

a) Record sites of injuries / contusions / pressure areas on Body Diagram below ☐

b) Record Waterlow Score - Waterlow Score: ....score

    Pressure Mattress   Given ☐   Not Applicable ☐
         Turn Hourly
         1Hour - Yes ☐   2 Hours – Yes ☐   Not Applicable ☐
    initial ....
    time   ....

Fig. 13.8. Extract from the Whittington Hospital Integrated Care Pathway for fractured neck of femur.

assessment, operation, recovery and rehabilitation. The ICP is used by all of the healthcare professionals involved, in place of their conventional records.

This ICP has now been in use for over 12 months, and has been well received. Many health professionals still repeat the same information on additional unstructured pages of clinical notes. It would appear that just recording their entries in several different parts of a large template, interleaved with entries of clinical colleagues, leaves a number of staff feeling that they have not completely expressed their findings and ideas.

Several studies have shown that computerised clinical record systems can improve clinician compliance with practice guidelines for preventive and active care.[55] Most evaluations of decision-support systems have been performed in the context of North American healthcare facilities and have been limited to measures of reliability, accuracy and acceptability.[56]

Where systems have been tested in the UK, this has often been in the context of outpatient clinics.[57] There has been little work on decision support within routine primary care consultations.[58,59]

The enactment of an electronic guideline and decision support function is of greatest clinical value when it is linked to the circumstances and needs of an individual patient. Guidelines therefore need to be linked with relevant individual clinical data-sets, in order to allow for their interactive use during patient encounters and by patients or their families at home. Existing paper-based guidelines will need to be expressed, formally, as flowcharts and algorithms in order to enable such an integration to occur. An appropriately expressed guideline would, for example, enable a clinical system to:

 accept a random blood glucose of 4.2 mmol/l

 warn the clinician when entering a blood glucose of 7.4 mmol/l, possibly invoking a textual message or initiating a protocol

reject a blood glucose of 74 mmol/l as a typing error.

It would be desirable if component software for implementing guidelines, from whatever source, could be interfaced to a wide range of EHCR products, including legacy systems and new products and systems to be developed in the future. To meet this objective, the electronic representation of clinical guidelines must meet three central requirements:

Seamlessness: between healthcare records systems, medical knowledge servers, and clinical decision support/guidelines systems.

Interoperability: facilitated by standardised clinical terminologies and codes, libraries of clinical protocols, and clinical data-sets.

Portability: the representation of the guidelines should be independent of the language in which it is expressed, the system on which it is implemented. It must embody communication standards such that it is capable of being shared between different sites.

Work is in progress on this challenge in the EU projects SynEx and Prompt.[49,50] It is anticipated that generic, system-independent, guidelines software products will be available within two years.

Audit, quality and behaviour change

The primary goal of clinical audit should be to foster a climate in which healthcare professionals collaborate to provide the highest quality of healthcare possible. Rather than focusing on the number and type of audits performed or on their findings, clinical governance should aim to promote a culture of working to standards and of encouraging clinicians to regularly review the quality of care they provide. It should promote a positive change in attitude within an organisation towards critical self-appraisal in the context of an open, supportive and learning environment. This should allow the obstacles to improving quality to be debated and successful ideas to be shared. Audit should not be a goal in itself or, worse still, simply a data collection exercise.

However, the additional data collection and analysis requirements of clinical audit are often obstacles to its performance. High quality clinical records are an invaluable resource with which to perform audit. Structured paper forms and computerised data-sets allow for the rapid aggregation of population data within or across healthcare organisations. Ideally, the commoner audit investigations should be automated as far as possible, to allow for regularly repeated quality reviews.

Clinicians are increasingly taking advantage of the opportunities the computer can offer to support the clinical consultation itself. Present-day systems have most frequently been used to collect more structured kinds of data, such as the reasons for encounters, chronic disease reviews and physiological measurements like blood pressure. Where such information has been entered methodically, doctors are already finding the electronic medical record an invaluable tool for reviewing patient summaries, for audit and for population analyses – see Figure 13.9.

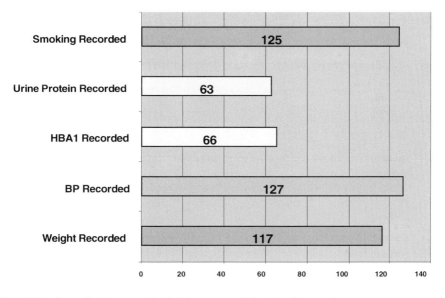

Fig. 13.9. An audit of computerised diabetes records in a London practice.

Clinical governance activities will require a more detailed analysis of clinical findings and actions than have hitherto been recorded in most computer systems. The expected future pattern of evolution of such systems has been discussed earlier in this chapter. In addition to the software tools required to review individual patient records, clinicians and managers will require more sophisticated query tools with which to group and interrogate records. These will need to present and compare overviews of performance and outcomes in ways that are readily understood by a wide range of professionals and by patients. These must be accepted as valid and it is important to recognise that data collected in this way must be analysed carefully.

It will be particularly important for clinical governance teams within an enterprise to recognise the sensitive nature of their work, and at the outset to develop a confidentiality policy that is enforced. Audit groups have recognised that many clinicians have a strong desire to improve on what they currently do, but a real lack of time and resources to identify and to implement the necessary changes. Changing professional behaviour requires a mixture of practical activities and often deep-seated shifts in approach that inevitably require personal education and support and time.

The support required by individuals and teams will vary enormously, and might include help to:

▶ identify appropriate topics for investigation

▶ agree on relevant and desirable standards

▶ design and perform audit methods

▶ analyse and discuss results obtained

▶ advise on the implementation of any appropriate changes

▶ identify and justify further resource needs for the team

▶ facilitate the provision of any necessary education and training.

Within this broad scope, individual audit activities should be undertaken in the light of a total quality approach to the care of each patient group. This might include:

▶ information about and access to a particular clinical service for patients and their families/carers

▶ the equipment, training and inter-working of the staff involved in providing care

▶ the use of protocols, evidence and other information resources (such as drug formularies)

▶ the complete recording of healthcare findings and activities, and the appropriate availability of this to relevant personnel at each point of care provision

▶ clinical and organisational audit, and other feedback mechanisms, to monitor overall quality

▶ critical event (clinical risk management) procedures to protect against serious error

▶ policies and procedures for staff appointment, appraisal, training and accreditation

▶ the safety and security of the environment for staff, patients and their information resources (e.g. patient records).

Ambitious teams will give consideration to formal quality assurance and organisational accreditation, such as that undertaken, in many sectors, under the umbrella of the ISO 9000 standard[60] or, in healthcare, through the Health Services Accreditation organisation[61] and The Kings Fund.[62,63]

Each organisation or team will need to consider the outcome and other measures of the services, which will be the basis for quality standards for audit. In this work, especially, it will need to work closely with patients and carers in order to focus on areas of healthcare in particular need of improvement; they often know best how the service fails to address their needs.

Data presentation and misrepresentation

The diversity of data-sets in daily use, in their various formats, is now at risk of becoming an obstacle to the improvement in the quality of shared care. Whilst providing the necessary framework to prompt authors to provide full information, anecdotal experience suggests that they are rather resented by those unfamiliar with them. Moreover, the time and effort required for a recipient of the data-set to navigate a structured template can sometimes be greater than that for scanning equivalent paragraphs of narrative text. Accident and emergency reports and post-natal discharge summaries are often quoted by general practitioners as examples of this.

There are no generic design principles to guide the definition or presentation of clinical data-sets. There is always a balance to be struck between structure and content within this structure, when expressing clinical concepts formally within records. Diversity of approach is inevitable, and even desirable, if forms are to serve specific local requirements of different groups, such as patients, institutions, specialties or professions. However, it does increase the complexity of record- and report-writing, and of record- or report-navigation, if a large number of such forms are in regular use and have a significant degree of overlap. It is often stated that electronic healthcare record systems with sophisticated browser tools will resolve this problem by allowing users to manipulate an unfamiliar data-set and represent it in their favourite way. Such tools might, for example, enable a diversity of styles of diabetes review entries within a single patient record, perhaps authored on different sites over time, to be presented in a uniform way.

In order to achieve this, in practical terms, healthcare record systems will need to support the clinician with clear and user-friendly screens, requiring a short data-entry time and providing a rapid display of past and recent health events. Summaries should be capable of customisation and provide an overview of family and psycho-social information. The full range of multi-media data types must be accessible.

Clinicians need help with using coded term sets. This should be made available from within data-entry templates and protocols, with user-friendly browsers and prompts and reminders to support good practice. Such browsing, prompting and analysis functions are already in use in some systems and are appreciated by users. But there are dangers in manipulating clinical facts and intentions without a rigorous record architecture and a comprehensive semantic formalism. Detaching part of a recorded entry from the original clinical context at the time that it was composed, carries the risk that it will be misinterpreted. The amalgamation of data which is inconsistent or from disparate sources easily leads to misleading or erroneous interpretations and conclusions.

Because clinical practice has historically endorsed the individuality of each patient and the personal style of each healthcare professional, combination of data-sets across patient records, even within a single department or general practice can prove quite a problem! The experience of Medical Audit Advisory Groups over recent years has demonstrated that even the use of common terminology can give rise to incompatible data sets.[64] Deriving meaningful information from aggregated data requires that the original data sets have been collected for a common purpose and in a consistent manner. It also requires that this purpose is known to the persons reviewing the aggregated data, when drawing their conclusions from it.

Ethical and legal issues

The ethical issues raised by the application of information technology to healthcare records are fundamentally important because there is a risk of serious harm to patients or to clinicians. However, the risk can be minimised without compromising the usefulness of the record, and regulation is both technically feasible and morally appropriate. Many of the ethical issues arise from the purposes of the healthcare record: the definition below was proposed by the GEHR project.[37]

▶ The primary purpose of the patient record is to benefit the patient by providing a record of care that supports present and future care by the same or other clinicians.

▶ The secondary purpose is to provide a medico-legal record of the care provided and hence support and demonstrate the competence of clinicians.

▶ Tertiary purposes must be legitimate (involve consent) and can never be allowed to compromise the primary or secondary purpose. Examples of tertiary purposes are the generation of data for health service management or public health programmes.

The foundations of the relationship between a clinician and a patient are the delivery of clinical care to the highest standard and the respect for patient autonomy. This inevitably means that the right to informed consent and the right to confidentiality are also moral principles of the highest importance behind a 'good' healthcare record system. Patients should exercise as much choice over the content and movement of their healthcare records as is consistent with good clinical care and the lack of serious harm to others. Records should be created, processed and managed in ways that optimally guarantee the confidentiality of their contents and legitimate control by patients in how they are used. The record must be secure yet accessible to patients. This strong patient focus is further developed and specified within the EU Directive on Data Protection.[24]

Clinical governance groups will need to recognise that the process of data aggregation for audit or other quality assurance activities inevitably takes individual clinical record entries out of their original context of recording. This creates the potential for misinterpretation and for breaching patient confidentiality.

The inappropriate disclosure of performance-related information to those outside the team or organisation also carries the risk of undermining professional morale and should be undertaken with knowledge and preferably with the consent of the clinical professionals involved. It is the experience of many audit facilitators that, on the occasions when audit has revealed outcomes that the individuals or groups involved themselves feel to be unsatisfactory, they are very astute in identifying the changes which need to be made, or will seek assistance in identifying and implementing appropriate changes. Formal procedures to rectify problem areas have rarely been required within a supportive and educational environment.

Data overload

Vastly more information is now gathered and is more easily available. It does not of itself improve the quality of care. Indeed forcing people to cope with too much information can increase the risk to patients.[65] Data and information overload will be a crucial issue in clinical governance. Both the growth in scientific literature and also working practices are equally responsible. The extent of the literature explosion can be illustrated by the facts that:[66]

▶ The learned literature has doubled every 10–15 years over the past 300 years.

▶ In the field of biomedicine 20,000 journals and 17,000 books are produced every year.

However the quality of the published literature is often very questionable. For instance three studies using consensus analysis by experts of published work on one topic showed that only 10–15% of articles were considered important.[67] The task of reviewing the literature, even with the support of information technology, is becoming increasingly more complex.[68] Although information technology has a role in managing the medical literature, it cannot 'cure' the rising volume. It has suggested, for example, that there should be some radical reforms, such as:

▶ Publish abstracts only; the full paper on request only.

▶ Limit papers to 50 per individual during career!

▶ Adopt more objective guidelines for judging quality.

The positive contributions that information technology can make in managing the medical literature are clear and becoming a practical reality. They include:

▶ A potential means of publishing, organising and communicating the literature.

▶ A personal window on the literature.

▶ A more efficient and effective means of access.

▶ A more economical use of time, for users and librarians.

There is the potential for the National Electronic Library for Health to play an important role in the organisation, accreditation and updating of clinical reference material. This service will become available on the NHSnet.

Education of healthcare professionals and their patients in the information age

A strategic and well-managed evolution towards complete and shared electronic healthcare records to enhance quality of care will require a considerable investment in both technical and educational resources. The levels of computer literacy amongst clinicians and managers are patchy. The training of personnel to use computers, clinical systems and medical knowledge systems will be a necessary component for the success of any clinical governance strategy. Surveys of healthcare staff demonstrate huge interest and willingness to improve skills and frustration at lack of time and resources within the working context to make this possible and worthwhile.[69]

A comprehensive set of electronic multi-media educational resources will be required to support consistent quality of care by clinicians and to empower patients to be contributors to their own healthcare. The design of such resources will need to include the indexing of topics with the content domain of healthcare records and with decision nodes of the protocols. The resources will need to be clustered into mini-tutorials to provide for educational themes targeted at a range of different knowledge levels, and grouped into a syllabus suitable for health professional learning and accreditation. Feedback loops will be required to allow for the evaluation of these materials and of the overall learning pathways taken by individuals and groups.

There are considerable educational implications of this potential information overload. The recommendations of the General Medical Council, in their document *Tomorrows Doctors* has begun to address this issue for the medical profession.[70] The principle recommendations include:

▶ The burden of factual information should be reduced.

▶ Learning through curiosity, the exploration of knowledge, and the critical evaluation of evidence should be promoted and should ensure a capacity for self-education.

▶ The undergraduate course should be seen as the first stage in the continuum of medical education that extends throughout professional life.

The opportunity for change in the delivery, the style, the content and the quality of education in the information age is huge.[71] It is also a threat to many established methods of education. Two quotations illustrate both the opportunities and the threats to current practice.

> So far as the mere imparting of information is concerned, no university has had any justification for existence since the popularisation of printing in the fifteenth century.[72]
>
> It is nothing short of a miracle that modern methods of instruction have not entirely strangled the holy curiosity of enquiry.[73]

Both Whitehead and Einstein might have approved of the use of information technology to seek to enrich the opportunities for learning, including perhaps the development of hyperbooks. Education, undergraduate, postgraduate and continuing is too large a subject for this chapter but it is so important for the future of the quality of healthcare.[74]

Leaflets, video and audio-tapes and more recently, computer programs have been seen as an integral part of a strategy designed to promote health, persuade people to adopt healthy lifestyles, and to increase the uptake of screening. They have also been used to help educate patients and their carers with certain chronic medical conditions. A lot of well-intentioned effort goes into producing this information. Unfortunately, the effort does not guarantee quality and usefulness. Information materials are no substitute for good verbal discussion, but there is a lot of evidence to demonstrate that consultations are usually so short that patients often do not obtain the information they want and need. Moreover, the patient's own data and information needs, in order to, for example, to take a decision about an intervention for breast cancer, may be very extensive.[75] They will want information about both risks and benefits of any intervention option. These sorts of needs are likely to increase with time, in both amount and sophistication.

Health-related websites are now available

Various checklists have been suggested to improve the quality and accuracy of health information.[76] In general, more attention has been paid to presentation and to readability than to content. The insistence on aiming for the lowest possible reading age may have contributed to the infantile quality of many materials. Meanwhile over 10,000 health-related websites are now available on the Internet. Much of the material is inaccurate or misleading.[77] Failure to address the quality of information obtained by patients will have serious consequences. Quality information, which the patient finds useful, is likely to enhance the quality and appropriateness of healthcare. The obverse will lead to inappropriate interventions, increased dissatisfaction and increased costs. There are strong arguments to establish an accreditation system, with appropriate evaluation, which will enable users to judge the quality of health information.[78] Users are, however, not uniform in their requirements; how can this be addressed?

A novel approach is being used in APoGI, an Internet database of information about the risks to children born to parents who are carriers of gene mutations which carry the risk of the haemoglobin disorder, thalassaemia. It combines the scientific knowledge about gene mutations and working from information provided by users, calculates the specific risks of possible outcomes in children born to the parents. The system also provides carefully designed essential information for all such parents, on the services they will need and the impact on them and their children of the conditions that may be inherited. As the presentation of advice is individually customised, a huge volume of potentially relevant material is filtered down to those parts essential in the current case. Moreover, the key scientific components of the database are the same the world over. A single database therefore can be developed, in this case by a WHO Collaborating Centre, and then made universally and practically instantaneously available. The whole content is evaluated and maintained within a world-wide community of patient support groups, counsellors and clinicians. The system (see Fig. 13.10) shows one approach to how information technology can assist in marrying a diverse body of knowledge to the specific needs of individuals. In this way they are led to high quality information that they require to meet their individual needs, without being 'swamped' with much unnecessary and confusing material. These issues are not so different in principle from those faced by the modern medical student.

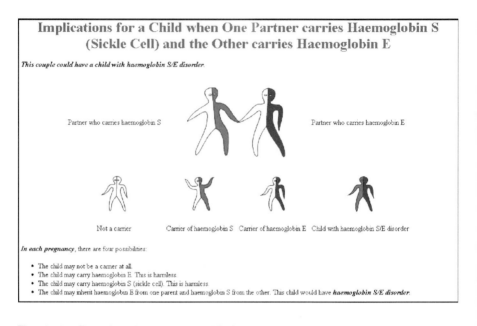

Fig. 13.10. Example web page from the APoGI resource.

Conclusions

Clinical governance is the start of a process. Its introduction is by far the most ambitious quality initiative that will ever have been implemented by the NHS.[79] To achieve its goals, it must facilitate change through concentration on the needs of those providing the service, through support and education, and on the building of new clinically-focused information systems. Information technology has many important roles in both these areas, in involving patients more fully in their self-management and providing tools to enable improvements in the quality of clinical care and education, at all levels of healthcare provision.

The potential of computers to support the administrative and financial management of hospitals and primary care practices is well recognised. Recent work within Europe has made significant progress in addressing the challenges of delivering the electronic healthcare record itself. Computer systems with the potential to capture, display and communicate a complete multi-media healthcare record are now becoming available. These are increasingly user-friendly, quick and intuitive to use and medico-legally sound. When clinical practice is able to adopt such EHCR systems, widely and as a realistic successor to the paper record, healthcare will be better supported in the challenges of providing integrated and seamless care, which is evidence-based and person-centred.

Medicine is an art as well as a science. If the computer can provide the tools necessary to enable healthcare professionals to practice scientifically and efficiently, clinicians should be better able to devote time and energy to the human side of their relationships with patients.

It may be appropriate to conclude with two apt quotations relevant to clinical governance. The first is from the person who probably invented it, **Florence Nightingale** in 1863, and demonstrates this is about all patients and professionals, not about doctors alone:

> In attempting to arrive at the truth, I have applied everywhere for information but in scarcely an instance have I been able to obtain hospital records fit for any purpose of comparison. If they could be obtained, they would enable us to decide many other questions besides the one alluded to. They would show subscribers how their money was being spent, what amount of good was really being done with it or whether the money was not doing mischief rather than good.

The second is from Burke, and emphasises the importance of maintaining perspective on what is currently done and what can realistically be achieved.

> . . . to lament the past, to conceive extravagant hopes of the future, are the common dispositions of the greatest part of mankind. **Edmund Burke** (1729–97), Thoughts on the causes of the present discontents.

References

1   The new NHS. Modern. Dependable. Cm 3807. December 1997.
2   Information for Health: An Information Strategy for the Modern NHS 1998.
3   Zimmerli W. Ch. Who has the right to know the genetic constitution of a particular person? In *Human Genetic Information: Science, Law and Ethics*, (Chadwick D, Bock G, Whelan T, Eds) J Wiley and Sons, Chichester, 1990.
4   Protti DJ. *The Synergism of Health Information Science/Health Informatics.* CRC Critical Reviews in Medical Informatics 1 part 2, 149–163, 1986.
5   Shortliffe EH. *http://camis.stanford.edu*
6   Technology Foresight: *Progress Through Partnership Vol 4*; Health and Life Sciences. HMSO Publications Centre, London.
7   Smith R. *The Future of Healthcare Systems.* BMJ 1997; 314: 1496–1496.
8   Deloitte & Touche. *Emerging trends in Information Technology.* MedInfo Conference Proceedings 8, Part 1, 1995.
9   Montgomery Hunter K. *Doctors Stories: The narrative structure of medical knowledge.* Princeton University Press, Princeton, New Jersey. 1991.
10 Southgate L, Berkson L and Fabb W et al. *Towards Better Definitions of Competence*: a Paper From the Cambridge Conference. Office of the Regius Professor of Medicine. Cambridge University. 1989.
11 Kalra D (ed.) The Synapses User Requirements and Functional Specification (Part A). *The Synapses Project.* Deliverable USER 1.1.1a. EU Telematics Application Programme Office, 1996.
12 Shortliffe EH and Barnett GO. *Medical Informatics: Computer Applications in Health Care.* Addison Wesley Publishing. Reading, Massachusetts. 1990.
13 McKay HG, Feil EG, Glasgow RE and Brown JE. *Feasibility and use of an internet support service for diabetes self-management.* Diabetes Educator 1998; 24: 174–179.
14 Carl F and Gribble TJ. HealthDesk for Haemophilia: an interactive computer and communications system for chronic illness self-management. Proceedings of the Annual Symposium on Computer Applications in Medical Care. 1995. AMIA, 1995: 829–833.
15 Bangemann M et al. Recommendations to the European Council: Europe and the global information society. Brussels: European Commission, 1994.
16 Drazen D. *Progress on Introducing the Computer Based Patient Record.* Conference Proceedings – Towards an Electronic Health Record Europe 1997. Medical Records Institute for the Centre for Advancement of Electronic Records Ltd. 1997; 74–84.

17   Blois M. Information and Medicine: *The Nature of Medical Descriptions*. Berkley and Los Angeles: University of California Press. 1984.

18   Rector A, Nowlan W and Kay S. *Methods of Informatics in Medicine*. 1991; 30: 179–186.

19   Derrett C, Kalra D and Gordon G. *Information and Information Systems in General Practice*: A Study in part of East London. Conference proceedings – Current Perspectives in Healthcare Computing 1996. BJHC Books. 1996; 716–717.

20   Audit Commission (UK), For Your Information – A Study of Information Management and Systems in Acute Hospitals. ISBN: 011 886 4165. HMSO Publications, London, 1995.

21   Smith R. *What Clinical Information do Doctors Need?* BMJ 1996; 313: 1062–1068.

22   Hearnshaw H, Baker R and Cooper A. A Survey of Audit Activity in General Practice. *British Journal of General Practice*, 1998; 48: 979–981.

23   The NHS IM&T Security Manual (IMG E5242). NHS Executive, Birmingham, England, 1996.

24   ENV 12924: Security Categorisation and Protection for Healthcare Information Systems. CEN TC/251, 1997. Brussels.

25   European Commission. European Union Directive 95/46/EC. On the protection of individuals with regard to the processing of personal data and on the free movement of such data. Brussels: European Commission, 1995.

26   Council of Europe Recommendation on the Protection of Medical Data, [R(97)5]. Brussels: European Commission, 1995.

27   Cimino J. *Bringing the Web to the Bed(side)*. Proceedings of IMIA International Working Conference on Electronic Patient Records in Medical Practice. 1998; 60–61.

28   Love B. *Developing National Standard Clinical EDI Messages*. In: Barahona P, Velosa M and Bryant J, eds. Conference Proceedings – Medical Informatics Europe 1994. Lisbon: European Federation for Medical Informatics, 1994.

29   O'Neill MJ, Payne C and Read JD. Read Codes Version 3: A User Led Terminology. Methods of Information in Medicine 1995; 34: 187–192.

30   Brennan S. The Electronic Patient Record Programme 1994–1996. Conference Proceedings – Towards an Electronic Health Record Europe 1996. Medical Records Institute for the Centre for Advancement of Electronic Records Ltd. 1996; 8–10.

31   Text of the Council Decision Adopting a Specific Programme of Research and Technological Development in the field of Communication Technologies, (1990–1994). Brussels 5/6/91.

32   Decision No. 1110/94/EC of the European Parliament and the Council, adopting a fourth framework programme of European Community activities in the field of research, technological development and demonstration (1994–1998).

33   Griffith SM, Kalra D, Lloyd DS and Ingram D. A Portable Communicative Architecture for Electronic Healthcare Records: the Good European Health Record Project. Medinfo 8 Part 1: 223–236, 1995.

34   Ingram D, Southgate L, Kalra D, Griffith S, Heard S et al. *GEHR Requirements for Clinical Comprehensiveness*. The Good European Health Record Project, Deliverable No. 4. AIM Office 1992.

35   Ingram D, Hap B, Lloyd D, Grubb P et al. *GEHR Requirements for Portability*. The Good European Health Record Project, Deliverable No. 5. AIM Office, 1992.

36   Ingram D, Lloyd D, Baille O, Grubb P et al. *GEHR Requirements for Communication Capacity*. The Good European Health Record Project, Deliverable No. 6. AIM Office, 1992.

37   Ingram D, Southgate L, Heard S, Doyle L, Kalra D et al. *GEHR Requirements for Ethical and Legal Acceptability*. The Good European Health Record Project, Deliverable No. 8. AIM Office, 1993.

38   Ingram D, Murphy J, Griffith S, Machado H et al. *GEHR Educational Requirements*. The Good European Health Record Project, Deliverable No. 9. AIM Office, 1993.

39   Hurlen P (ed.). ENV 12265: Electronic Healthcare Record Architecture. CEN TC/251 PT 1–011. Brussels, 1995.

40   A CORBA-based integration of distributed electronic healthcare records using the Synapses approach, J Grimson, W Grimson, D Berry, D Kalra, P Toussaint and O Weier. Special Issue of IEEE Transactions on Information Technology in Biomedicine on Emerging Health Telematics Applications In Europe, Vol 2, No 3; 124–138. 1998.

41   Kalra D (ed.). *Synapses ODP Information Viewpoint*. The Synapses Project. EU Telematics Application Programme Office, 1998.

42   Rector A, Zanstra P, Solomon D and The GALEN Consortium (1995). GALEN: Terminology Services for Clinical Information Systems in Health in the New Communications Age. M. Laires, M. Ladeira and J. Christensen (ed). Amsterdam, IOS Press. 90–100.

43   O'Neill MJ and Brown PJ. *Why Headings Need a Model*. Internal Working Paper, NHS Centre for Coding and Classification. February 1997.

44   Severs M et al. *Headings for Communicating the Personal Health Record.* NHS Executive, 1997.

45   Rossi Mori A et al. Electronic Health Care Record Communication: Part 2 – Domain Termlist – First Working Document (PT27 – N13). CEN TC/251, Brussels, 1998.

46   Barber B et al. *Data security for health care.* SEISMED Consortium – Studies in Health Technology and Informatics. Amsterdam: IOS Press, 1996. ISBN: 90 5199 263 7 (three vols.)

47   Barber B et al. *Towards security in medical telematics: Legal and Technical Aspects.* SEISMED Consortium – Studies in Health Technology and Informatics. Amsterdam: IOS Press, 1996: 27. ISBN: 90 5199 246 7.

48   Source: http://ted.see.plym.ac.uk/ishtar/

49   Kalra D, Austin A, Ingram D, Patterson D, Ferrara F, Sottille P, Grimson W and Solomon D. *The SynEx Project.* Conference Proceedings – Towards an Electronic Health Record Europe 1998. Medical Records Institute for the Centre for Advancement of Electronic Records Ltd. 1998; 290–297.

50   Lagouarde P, Thomson R, Renaud-Salis JL, Ferguson P, Hajnal S and Robles P, The PROMPT Electronic Health Care Record in Brender J, Christensen J P, Scherrer J-R McNair P (eds) Medical Informatics Europe 1996 IOS Press, Amsterdam 1996, pp. 1055–1059.

51   Source: http://www.centc251.org/

52   Field M and Lohr K, eds. *Clinical practice guidelines:directions for a new program.* Washington: National Academy Press, 1990.

53   Haines A and Feder G. *Guidance on guidelines: writing them is easier than making them work.* BMJ 1992; 305: 785–786.

54   Grimshaw JM and Russell IT. *Do explicit guidelines change medical practice?* A systematic review of rigorous evaluations. Lancet 1993; 342: 1317–1322.

55   Johnston ME, Langton KB, Haynes RB and Mathieu A. Effects of computer-based clinical decision support systems on clinician performance and patient outcome: a critical appraisal of research. Ann Int Med 1994; 120: 135–142.

56   Barnett GO. *The Application of Computer-Based Medical-Record Systems in Ambulatory Practice.* N Engl J Med 1984; 310: 1643–1650.

57   Lilford R, Kelly M and Baines A. *Effect of using protocols on medical care: randomised trial of three methods of taking an antenatal history.* British Medical Journal 1992; 305: 1181–1183.

58   Purves IN. Prodigy Interim Report. Journal of Informatics in Primary Care 1996; (Sept): 2–8.

59   Wyatt JC. *Use and Sources of Medical Knowledge.* Lancet 1991; 338: 1368–1373.

60   Quality Management and Quality Assurance Standards. ISO 9000: 1991. Geneva, Switzerland.

61   Service Standards Reports (series). Health Services Accreditation, Rutherford Park, Marley Lane, Battle, East Sussex TN33 0EZ. http://www.nhs-accreditation.co.uk

62   Organisational Audit (Accreditation UK): Standards for an Acute Hospital. King's Fund Centre, 1990.

63   Organisational Audit (Accreditation UK): Standards of Primary Health Care. King's Fund Centre, 1993.

64   Source: Camden & Islington and East London & the City Medical Audit Advisory Groups.

65   Vincent C (Ed). *Clinical Risk Management.* BMJ Publishing Group, 1995.

66   Shortliffe EH, Perrault LE. *Medical Informatics: Computer Applications in Health Care.* Addison-Wesley, USA 1990.

67   Goffman W. *The Ecology of the Biomedical Literature and Information Retrieval.* In: Warren S, ed. Coping with the biomedical literature. Praeger, New York 1981.

68   Lock S. *Information overload: solution by quality?* BMJ 1982; 284: 1289–90.

69   Murphy J, Errington R, Achara S, Simon R and Olaiwon (1997). Preparing the Next Generation of Clinicians to Manage Information, in Pappas C, Maglaveras N and Scherrer J-R (eds), Medical Informatics Europe 1997, IOS Press, pp. 676–680.

70   Tomorrows Doctors: *Recommendations on Undergraduate Medical Education.* General Medical Council, London 1993.

71   MacFarlane AGJ (Ed) *Teaching and Learning in an Expanding Higher Education System. Report of a working party of the Committee of Scottish University Principals.*

72   Whitehead AN cited by West K. *The case against teaching.* J Med Educ 1996; 41: 766–771.

73   Einstein A cited by West K. J Med Educ 1996; 41: 766–771.

74   Jolly B, Rees L, Eds. *Medical Education in the Millenium.* Oxford Medical Publications, 1998.

75   Pierce PF. *Deciding on breast cancer treatment: a description of decision behaviour.* Nursing Research 1993; 42: 22–28.

76   checklists for content of health information sheets

77   Wyatt JC. *Measuring quality and impact of the World Wide Web.* BMJ 1997 314: 1879–1881.

78   Coulter A. *Evidence based patient information.* BMJ 1998 317: 225–226.

79   Scally G and Donaldson IJ. *Clinical governance and the drive for quality improvement in the new NHS in England.* BMJ 1998; 317: 61–65.

▶14

Guide to Sources

Rosemary Hittinger, Julie Glanville, Jane Cartwright, Sue Johnson, Dorothy Gregson

Clinical Audit

*The systematic and critical analysis of the quality of clinical care, including the procedures used for diagnosis, treatment and care, the associated use of resources and the resulting outcomes and quality of life for the patient.***Working For Patients 1989**.
  Clinical Audit is a multi-disciplinary activity which uses peer evaluation to demonstrate and improve the quality of patient care.

Organisations:
Association for Quality in Healthcare
Clinical Audit is only one of the special interest/focus groups provided by this organisation which was established to bring together individuals and organisations who have an interest in continuously improving the quality of healthcare in the UK and in furthering the knowledge related to the subject of quality in healthcare. To promote measurable and continuous improvement in the quality of healthcare for the benefit of the public. Also working to provide professional recognition of healthcare workers with specific responsibility for quality matters. Provides:

▶ regular Journal (recently re-launched as *Healthcare Quality*)

▶ regular branch/special interest meetings

▶ educational programme.

Association for Quality in Healthcare,	**Tel:** 01962 8777000
47 Southgate Street,	**Fax:** 01962 877701
Winchester	
Hants SO23 9EH	

Clinical Audit Association
First professional audit organisation established 1991 to provide support for healthcare professionals working in this field and to provide a focus for the development and promotion of clinical audit in the UK. Was responsible for pioneering work on systematic identification of occupational standards for healthcare professionals working in this field. Provides:

▶ regular newsletter 'Network'

▶ flexible learning programme leading to National Certificate in Clinical Audit.

Clinical Audit Association Ltd.,
Cleethorpes Business Centre,
Jackson Place,
Wilton Road,
Humberston,
North East Lincolnshire
DN36 4AS

Tel/Fax 01472 210682
email: pmkent@the-caa-ltd.demon.co.uk
website: http://www.the-caa-ltd.demon.co.uk

National Centre for Clinical Audit

Government funded body established June 1995 to facilitate best practice in healthcare by promoting multi disciplinary clinical audit. Provides:

- information
- advice & support
- standards for excellence in clinical audit
- database of audit projects
- educational events and conferences
- regular newsletter.

National Centre for Clinical Audit
BMA House
Tavistock Square
London WC1H 9JP

Tel: 0171 383 6451
Fax: 0171 383 6373
email: NCCA@ncca.org.uk
website:http://www.ncca.org.uk

WEB SITE: Very useful interactive website providing a wide range of services. Full access available on registration.

Scottish Clinical Audit Resource Centre

Established in 1994 to promote education and communication between different workers in the NHS in Scotland, to facilitate information sharing, better understanding and improved clinical care. Twice yearly newsletter produced. Work of the Centre includes:

- education and training courses
- information Services. Library and Audit Project register
- research; audit and clinical effectiveness, implementation of clinical guidelines etc.

Scottish Clinical Audit Resource
Centre,
Glasgow University,
1 Horselethill Road,
Glasgow G12 9LX

Tel: 0141 330 6190
Fax: 0141 330 6192
email: SCARC@pgm.gla.ac.uk
website:
http://info.gla.ac.uk.Acad/PGMed/SCARC

Audit (and associated) Activities of the Royal Colleges and their Faculties in the UK

Not all of the Royal Colleges and their associated bodies have identified audit departments. Department names and contact addresses are shown where appropriate.

Royal College of Anaesthetists

Quality of Practice Committee,
Royal College of Anaesthetists,
48–49 Russell Square,
LONDON WC1B 4JY

Tel: 0171 813 1900
Fax: 0171 813 1876
website: http://www.rcoa.ac.uk/

Co-ordinates national audits, produces and disseminates guidelines, has a professional standards committee.

Royal College of General Practitioners

Effective Clinical Practice Unit,
University of Sheffield,
Regent Court,
30 Regent House,
Sheffield S1 4DA

Tel: 0114 222 0811

Produces clinical practice guidelines and is developing a national quality clinical practice programme. Also see following entry.

Royal College of General Practitioners

Guidelines Initiative and Quality
Network,
14 Princes Gate,
Hyde Park,
London SW7 1PU

Tel: 0171 581 3232 ext 242
Fax: 0171 225 3047
email: pmmcdowell@regp.org.uk/
        fzwanenberg@regp.org.uk

Provides a service to GPs and partner organisations co-ordinating and disseminating guidelines, etc. Is a division of the Effective Clinical Practice Unit based at the University of Sheffield. See previous entry.

Royal College of Obstetricians & Gynaecologists

Audit Unit,
St Mary's Hospital,
Hathersage Road,
Whitworth Park,
Manchester M13 0JH

Tel: 0161 276 6300
Fax: 0161 276 6311

Royal College of Paediatrics & Child Health

Audit Unit,
Royal College of Paediatrics &
Child Health,
50 Hallam Street,
London W1N 6DR

Tel: 0171 307 5674
Fax: 0171 307 5679
email: research@rcpch.ac.uk

Maintains comprehensive databases: clinical audit projects, clinical guidelines. Co-ordinates national audits and active in clinical guideline development in specific fields. Has produced an extremely useful guide to Internet Sites.

Royal College of Pathologists

Clinical Audit Unit,
2 Carlton House Terrace,
London SW1Y 5AF

Tel: 0171 930 5864
Fax: 0171 321 0523
email: 106235.1777@compuserve.com

Royal College of Physicians

Research Unit,
11 St Andrew's Place,
Regent's Park,
London NW1 4LE

Tel: 0171 935 0332
Fax: 0171 487 3988
email: luna.islam@rcplondon.ac.uk

Audit and guideline activity is co-ordinated from this Unit.

Royal College of Radiologists

Clinical Audit Adviser,
38 Portland Place,
London W1N 4JQ

Tel: 0171 436 4251
Fax: 0171 323 3100
email: enquiries@rcr.ac.uk

Sets standards for members' participation in audit activity, disseminates guidelines and issues a guide for others to make the best use of a department of radiology.

Royal College of Surgeons of England

Surgical Epidemiology & Audit Unit,
Royal College of Surgeons of England,
35/43 Lincoln's Inn Fields,
London WC2A 3PN

Tel: 0171 405 3474
Fax: 0171 831 5741
web site:
http:/www/grhlib.demon.co.uk/
rcsaudit.html

Actively promotes audit activity of its members by making participation in audit meetings a mandatory requirement for the educational approval of surgical training posts. Produces and disseminates guidelines both on conduct of audit activity and specific disease management.

Royal College of Surgeons of England

Comparative Audit Service,   **Tel:** 0171 973 2166
Royal College of Surgeons of England,   **Fax:** 0171 831 5741
35/43 Lincoln's Inn Fields,
London WC2A 3PN

Set up in 1990 to provide Consultants with a better understanding of their practice and how it compares with others. Designed to be non-judgemental and to help identify areas where local audit activity should be undertaken. **The Comparative Patient Satisfaction Service** is complementary to this function.

Centrally Funded National Audits

Audit of Intensive Care and High Dependency Care

Intensive Care National Audit &   **Tel:** 0171 388 2856
  Research Centre (ICNARC);   **Fax:** 0171 388 3759
Tavistock House   **email:** Kathy@icnarc.demon.co.uk
Tavistock Square,
London WC1H 9HR

Confidential Enquiry into Suicide & Homicide by People with Mental Illness

PO Box 86,   **Tel:** 0161 291 4751/4752
Manchester M20 2EF   **Fax:** 0161 291 4358

Confidential Enquiries into Maternal Deaths (CEMD)

Room 729,   **Tel:** 0171 972 4344
Wellington House,   **Fax:** 0171 972 4348
135–155 Waterloo Road,
London SE1 8UG

Confidential Enquiries into Stillbirths & Deaths in Infancy (CESDI)

Chiltern Court,   **Tel:** 0171 486 1191
188 Baker Street,   **Fax:** 0171 486 6543
London NW1 5SD   **email:** admin@cesdi.org.uk

Confidential Enquiries into Counselling for Genetic Disorders

Genetic Enquiry Centre,   **Tel:** 0161 276 6262
6th Floor,   **Fax:** 0161 248 8308
St Mary's Hospital,   **email:** rodney.harris@man.ac.uk
Manchester

National Clinical Audit of Hospital Infection Control

Central Public Health Laboratory,	**Tel:** 0181 200 4400
Laboratory of Hospital Infection,	**Fax:** 0181 200 7449
61 Colindale Avenue,	
London NW9 5HT	

National Comparative Audit

Royal College of Surgeons of England,	**Tel:** 0171 405 3474
35/43 Lincoln's Inn Fields,	**Fax:** 0171 831 9483
London WC2A 3PN	

National Confidential Enquiry into Peri-operative Deaths (NCEPOD)

35–43 Lincoln's Inn Fields,	**Tel:** 0171 831 6430
London WC2A 3PN	**Fax:** 0171 430 2958

National Confidential Enquiry into Interventional Radiology

see above

UK Trauma Audit & Research Network

Clinical Sciences Building,	**Tel:** 0161 787 4397
University of Manchester,	**Fax:** 0161 787 4345
Hope Hospital,	**email:** maralynw@fslho.man.ac.uk
Salford,	dyates@fslho.man.ac.uk
Manchester M6 8HD	

Journals and/or Periodicals

The following are a list of publications with a primarily audit emphasis. There are many other publications concentrating on general healthcare quality matters which are not included here.

Audit Trends

Eli Lilly National Clinical Audit Centre,	**Tel:** 0116 258 4873
Department of General Practice,	
University of Leicester,	
Leicester General Hospital,	
Gwendolen Road,	
Leicester LE5 4PM	

Network
Newsletter of the Clinical Audit
Association
Clinical Audit Association Ltd.,   **Tel/Fax:** 01472 210682
Cleethorpes Business Centre,
Jackson Place,
Wilton Road,
Humberston,
North East Lincolnshire
DN36 4AS

Journal of Evaluation in Clinical Practice
Blackwell Science Ltd.,
Osney Mead,
Oxford
OX2 0EL

Healthcare Quality
Journal of the Association for Quality
in Healthcare
DP Media (Head Office),   **Tel:** 0171 976 1977
9 Irving Street,
Leicester Square,
London WC2H 7AT

Quality in Healthcare
Subscription Manager,
Quality in Healthcare,
BMJ Publishing Group,
PO Box 299,
London WC1H 9TD

Courses
Since clinical (originally medical) audit was first identified as a mandatory quality assurance activity in healthcare in 1989 a number of courses have been developed to enhance the professional development of those working in this field. Some of these courses now result in a recognised professional qualification. The following list is by no means exhaustive as new ones are being developed all the time.

National Certificate in Clinical Audit
Newly (1998) established flexible learning programme aimed at enabling those who have been working in the field of clinical audit to gain a recognised qualification utilising their existing experience and work.

Patricia Kent,
Clinical Audit Association Ltd.,
Cleethorpes Business Centre,
Jackson Place,
Wilton Road,
Humberston,
North East Lincolnshire
DN36 4AS

Tel/Fax: 01472 210682
email: pmkent@the-caa-ltd.demon.co.uk

Certificate in Medical and Clinical Audit
First professional qualification established in audit. Designed for experienced audit staff who are keen to enhance skills.

School of Postgraduate Studies in
   Medical & Healthcare,
University of Wales,
Morriston Hospital,
Swansea SA6 6NL

Tel: 01792 703578
Fax: 01792 797310
email: pmschool@swansea.ac.uk

MSc in Clinical Audit and Effectiveness
Course aimed to provide the knowledge, skills and understanding necessary for a healthcare professional to promote, support and/or undertake evidence based clinical practice.

School of Postgraduate Studies in
   Medical & Healthcare,
University of Wales,
Morriston Hospital,
Swansea SA6 6NL

Tel: 01792 703578
Fax: 01792 797310
email: pmschool@swansea.ac.uk

MSc in Evaluation of Clinical Practice
Two year part time day-release course leading to MSc degree or one year day release course leading to a diploma.

University of Westminster,
115 New Cavendish Street,
London W1M 8JS

Tel: 0171 911 5883
Fax: 0171 911 5079
email: cavadmin@wmin.ac.uk

Basic Audit Training
Three day foundation course for those new to clinical audit.

PMK Training Associates,	**Tel:** 01472 813258
25 Westport Road,	**Fax:** 01472 813258
Cleethorpes,	
North Lincolnshire DN35 0QF	

Please note PMK Training Associates also provide a number of courses to develop and enhance the skills required by audit professionals such as questionnaire design, interview techniques, statistics, etc. Further details from the above address.

Introduction to Clinical Audit
Three day foundation course for those new to clinical audit.

Eli Lilly National Clinical Audit Centre,	**Tel:** 0116 258 4873
Department of General Practice and	
Primary Care,	
University of Leicester,	
Leicester General Hospital,	
Leics LE5 4PW	

Certificate in Clinical Audit Support

Eli Lilly National Clinical Audit Centre,	**Tel:** 0116 258 4873
Department of General Practice and	
Primary Care,	
University of Leicester,	
Leicester General Hospital,	
Leics LE5 4PW	

Using Clinical Audit to Improve Clinical Effectiveness
Five day course for those supporting clinical audit and clinical effectiveness programmes.

Healthcare Quality Quest,	**Tel:** 01703 814024
Shelley Farm,	**Fax:** 01703 814020
Shelley Lane,	**email:** HQQ.co.uk
Ower,	
Romsey,	
Hants SO51 6AS	

'Advanced' course available as well as a one day critical appraisal workshop. Consultancy service also provided to independently review in-house audit departments. Further details from the above address.

Clinical effectiveness

The concept that healthcare treatments should be effective and cost-effective, and that evidence on the effectiveness of treatments should be sought from well conducted research. Clinical effectiveness involves assessing the research evidence to determine whether interventions work, presenting the findings on what is most effective and disseminating those findings to encourage changes in practice. Information on the clinical effectiveness of interventions tends to come from systematic reviews of primary studies, and may be disseminated in a variety of formats.

The following list of key organisations, programmes and information resources is necessarily selective and is biased towards the UK.

Organisations

Aggressive Research Intelligence Facility (ARIF)

An initiative funded by the West Midlands Regional Office to provide support to purchasers in finding and interpreting research evidence to inform decisions. The summaries of ARIFs findings on specific effectiveness questions are available on the Internet.

27 Highfield Road, **Tel/Fax:** 0121 455 6852
Edgbaston,   **email:** c.j.hyde@bham.ac.uk
Birmingham B15 3DP **website:** http://www.hsrc.org.uk/links/arif/arifhome.htm

Agency for Health Care Policy and Research (AHCPR)

This US agency conducted a series of large scale reviews in the mid 1990s which are available full text on the Internet. They are now commissioning evidence reports 'based on comprehensive reviews and rigorous analyses of the relevant scientific evidence'.

Agency for Health Care Policy and Research, **email:** info@ahcpr.gov
Executive Office Center, Suite 400,   **website:** http://text.nlm.nih.gov/
2101 East Jefferson Street,
Rockville, MD 20852, USA

Cochrane Collaboration

A world-wide network of researchers producing methodologically rigorous systematic reviews of the effectiveness of healthcare interventions based primarily on assessments of the evidence from randomised controlled trials. The reviews are published as the Cochrane Database of Systematic Reviews, which is available as part of the Cochrane Library (a CD-ROM based collection of databases which has also recently been launched on the World Wide Web). The Collaboration also compiles the Cochrane Controlled Trials Register: a unique collection of 200,000 controlled clinical trials (the raw material for many systematic reviews).

Information on the Cochrane Collaboration:

UK Cochrane Centre,	**Tel:** 01865 516300
Summertown Pavilion,	**Fax:** 01865 516311
Middle Way,	**email:** general@cochrane.co.uk
Oxford OX2 7LG	**website:** http://www.imbi.uni-freiburg.de/cochrane/

Information on the Cochrane Library:

Update Software,	**Tel:**01865 513902
PO Box 696,	**Fax:** 01865 516918
Oxford OX2 7YX	**email:** update@cochrane.co.uk
	website: http://www.update-software.com/ccweb/cochrane/cdsr.htm

Health Evidence Bulletins – Wales

These bulletins summarise the research evidence on key questions across broad categories of healthcare such as maternal and early child health. The sources of evidence are clearly referenced and reports are available in full on the Internet.

Duthie Library,	**Tel:** 01222 745142
University of Wales College of Medicine,	**Fax:** 01222 743651
Cardiff	**email:**
CF4 4XN	weightmanal@cardiff.ac.uk
	website:
	http://www.uwcm.ac.uk/uwcm/lb/pep/index.html

NHS Centre for Reviews and Dissemination (CRD)

Funded by the UK Departments of Health to provide information on the effectiveness and cost-effectiveness of healthcare interventions and ways of organising healthcare. CRD carries out systematic reviews and publishes evidence-based summaries and patient leaflets. CRD's reviews frequently use evidence from study designs other than randomised controlled trials. It promotes access to other sources of clinical effectiveness information by producing databases and providing training in how to search the Cochrane Library. The Centre also disseminates the results of reviews in innovative ways. Its main products are:

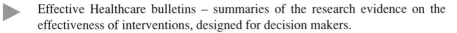 Effective Healthcare bulletins – summaries of the research evidence on the effectiveness of interventions, designed for decision makers.

Effectiveness Matters – brief bulletins on key messages from research.

Database of Reviews of Abstracts of Effectiveness (DARE) – critical summaries of quality assessed published systematic reviews.

NHS Economic Evaluation Database – critical summaries of economic evaluations of healthcare interventions.

 Technology Assessment Database – author abstracts of technology assessment reports published by agencies around the world.

 Patient and practitioner leaflets – based on research evidence.

NHS Centre for Reviews and Dissemination, University of York, York YO1 5DD	**Tel:** 01904 433707 **Fax:** 01904 433661 **email:** revdis@york.ac.uk **website:** http://www.york.ac.uk/inst/crd

NHS Health Technology Assessment Programme

This programme prioritises and commissions research of importance to the NHS, which may include systematic reviews as well as primary research. The research results are published as Technology Assessment Reports and are available in print and on the Internet.

Programme Manager's Office, National Co-ordinating Centre for Health Technology Assessment, Mailpoint 728, Boldrewood, University of Southampton, Highfield, Southampton SO16 7PX	**Tel:** 01703 595586 **Fax:** 01703 595639 **email:**hta@soton.ac.uk **website:** http://www.soton.ac.uk/.hta/htapubs.htm

Scottish Health Purchasing Information Centre (SHPIC)

A Scottish initiative to carry out and commission systematic reviews to inform health purchasing decisions in Scotland. Its reports are available in print and on the Internet.

SHPIC, Summerfield House, 2 Eday Road, Aberdeen AB15 6RE	**Tel:** 01224 663456 **website:** http://www.nhsconfed.net/shpic/

Scottish Intercollegiate Guidelines Network (SIGN)

This network compiles guidelines based on research evidence.

SIGN Administrative Support Centre, Royal College of Physicians, 9 Queen Street, Edinburgh EH2 1JQ	**Tel:** 0131 225 7324 **Fax:** 0131 220 4393 **email:** r.harbour@rcpe.ac.uk **website:** http://pc47.cee.hw.ac.uk/sign/home.htm

US Preventive Services Task Force

Produce guidelines supplying research-based evidence on the effectiveness of preventive health strategies: Guide to Clinical Preventive Services. 2nd ed. Baltimore: Williams and Wilkins, 1996. (ISBN: 0–683–08508–5). The guide is also available on the Internet.

website: http://text.nlm.nih.gov/

Databases

Best Evidence

A CD-ROM product containing the full text of the two journals: *ACP Journal Club* and *Evidence-Based Medicine*. These journals offer critical summaries of published research.

BMJ Publishing Group,	**Tel:** 0171 383 6270
PO Box 299,	**Fax:** 0171 383 6402
London WC1H 9TD	

Cochrane Database of Systematic Reviews

See Organisations: Cochrane Collaboration

Cochrane Library

See Organisations: Cochrane Collaboration

Database of Abstracts of Reviews of Effectiveness

See Organisations: NHS Centre for Reviews and Dissemination

Evidence-Based Medicine Reviews (EBMR)

A recently launched database combining and linking the Cochrane Database of Systematic Reviews and Best Evidence, to MEDLINE.

website: http://www.ovid.com/

NHS Economic Evaluation Database

See Organisations: NHS Centre for Reviews and Dissemination

Journals

ACP Journal Club

This journal offers critical appraisals of primary research (such as randomised controlled trials and economic evaluations) and systematic reviews with a commentary from a clinical expert. The journal is also available on *Best Evidence* (See: Databases).

website: http://www.acponline.org/journals/acpjc/jcmenu.htm

Bandolier
Articles about the clinical effectiveness of interventions and ways of interpreting the research evidence. Available in print and full text on the Internet:

Hayward Medical Communications,   **Tel:** 01865 226132
Rosemary House,   **Fax:** 01865 226978
Lanwades Park,   **website:**
Kentford,   http://www.jr2.ox.ac.uk:80/Bandolier
near Newmarket,
Suffolk CB8 7PW

Drug and Therapeutics Bulletin
This journal reviews drugs and is aimed at UK general practitioners and pharmacists. It is available in print and on the British National Formulary CD-ROM.

Dept. DTB,   **Tel:** 01992 822800
Consumers' Association,   **website:** http://www.which.net
Castlemead,
Gascoyne Way,
Hertford SG14 1LH

Effective Healthcare Bulletins
See Organisations: NHS Centre for Reviews and Dissemination

Effectiveness Matters
See Organisations: NHS Centre for Reviews and Dissemination

Evidence-Based Medicine
Critical appraisals of primary research (such as randomised controlled trials and economic evaluations) and systematic reviews with a commentary from a clinical expert. The journal is also available on *Best Evidence* (See: Databases).

BMJ Publishing Group,   **Tel:** 0171 383 6270
PO Box 299,   **Fax:** 0171 383 6402
London WCIH 9TD

Journal of Clinical Effectiveness
Publishes papers on evidence-based practice, clinical effectiveness, guidelines and audit and aims to be 'practical and clinically-based'.

Financial Times Professional Ltd.,   **Tel:** 0800 801 405
PO Box 77,
Subscriptions (Journals) Department,
Harlow,
Essex CM19 5BQ

Indexes to Clinical Effectiveness Resources

Clinical effectiveness information is published in a variety of formats, many of which are not recorded by major databases such as MEDLINE, which tend to concentrate on journal articles. The following Internet resources index many, but not all, of the key clinical effectiveness publications available on the WWW and offer searching by subject.

TRIP
Produced by the Turning Research Into Practice (TRIP) initiative in Gwent.
website: http://www.gwent.nhs.gov.uk/trip/test-search.html

ScHARR-Lock's Guide to the Evidence
Produced by Andrew Booth of the School of Health and Related Research, University of Sheffield.
website:http://www.shef.ac.uk/uni/ academic/R-Z/scharr/ir/scebm.html

Guides to Clinical Effectiveness Resources

Booth A.
The ScHARR guide to evidence-based practice. Sheffield: University of Sheffield, School of Health and Related Research, 1997. (Occasional Paper 97/2)

NHS Executive Public Health Development Unit.
Clinical effectiveness. Resource pack. [London]: Department of Health, 1997. Available from: NHS responseline: **Tel:** 0541 555 455 (catalogue number 97CC115).

Programmes Investigating the Implementation of Clinical Effectiveness Information

Evaluation of methods to promote the implementation of research findings
Programme of research co-ordinated by the North Thames Regional Office.

Melanie Baillie-Johnston,
National R&D Commissioning Unit
   (North Thames),
R&D Directorate,
40 Eastbourne Terrace,
London W2 3QR

Tel: 0171 725 5395
Fax: 0171 725 5467
email: mjohnsop@doh.gov.uk

website: http://www.open.gov.uk/doh/ntrd/rd/implem/index.htm

Framework for Appropriate Care Throughout Sheffield (FACTS)
c/o ScHARR,   **Tel:** 0114 275 5658
Regent Court,   **Fax:** 0114 275 5653
30 Regent Street,   **email:** Facts@Sheffield.ac.uk
Sheffield S1 4DA
website: http://www.shef.ac.uk/uni/projects/facts

Promoting Action on Clinical Effectiveness (PACE)
A series of projects on turning research into practice co-ordinated by the King's Fund.

The King's Fund,   **Tel:** 0171 307 2400
11–13 Cavendish Square,   **Fax:** 0171 307 2801
London   **email:** web@kehf.org.uk
W1M 0AN
website: http://www.kingsfund.org.uk/pace/evidence.htm

ARIF
See Organisations: Aggressive Research Intelligence Function

TRIP
See: Indexes To Clinical Effectiveness Resources

Clinical Risk Management

'Clinical risk management is a mechanism for managing exposure to risk that enables us to recognise the damaging consequences in the future, their severity and how they can be controlled.' Dickson G, *Principles of Risk Management*, quality in Healthcare 1995; 4: 75–79.

Organisations:

ALARM (Association of Litigation and Risk Management)
Objectives/Activities:

 To improve patient care by promoting effective risk management.

 To cut the cost of litigation by encouraging best practice in the investigation and management of claims.

 To provide a forum for risk and claims managers to share experiences, exchange information and develop solutions to clinical risk and claims management problems.

Membership is corporate and named representatives are responsible for managing clinical negligence claims and the implementation of clinical risk management programmes.

Three seminars per year are held in London and a Newsletter is produced for members. There are also regular training courses in relevant topics.

Contact: Jane Chapman,
ALARM,
1 Wimpole Street,
London,
W1M 8AE
Tel: 0171 290 2968
Fax: 0171 290 2989

Chesterfield Clinical Risk Management Group
Contact: Brian Gibbs,
Director of Support Services,
Bassetlaw Hospital and Community Services NHS Trust,
Bassetlaw District General Hospital,
Kilton,
Worksop,
S81 OBD,
Tel: 01909 500990
Fax: 01909 502810

CNST (Clinical Negligence Scheme for Trusts)
Objectives/Activities:

▶ Setting and auditing of clinical risk management standards for member Trusts.

▶ Issuing periodical newsletter and guidance.

▶ Roadshows to raise awareness and knowledge.

Contact: Roger Mason,
Risk Management Co-ordinator,
Howard House,
Queens Avenue,
Bristol,
BS8 1SN
Tel: 0117 926 2091
Fax: 0117 929 9845

Assessors: Sarah Hepworth (North of England) 0191 253 5623
Wendy Huxley Marko (Midlands) 0156 879 7667
Caroline Brown (South of England) 0196 285 6940

Clinical Risk Unit

The Clinical Risk Unit (CRU) was established in April 1995 with funding from the North Thames Health Agencies to continue and develop the North West Thames risk management project. The CRU has focused on two main functions: (i) to design and run the North Thames training programme in risk management and (ii) to carry out research into the cause and consequences of injury to patients, complaints and litigation and to develop effective methods of prevention.

For information on research Contact:

        Charles Vincent,
        Director of the Clinical Risk Unit,
        Psychology Dept,
        Clinical Risk Unit,
        1–19 Torrington Place,
        University College London,
        Gower Street,
        London,
        WCIE 6BT
        Tel: 0171 504 5948
        Fax: 0171 391 1647
        email:c.vince@ucl.ac.uk

See Training section for contacts for CRU courses.

Health Services Management Centre (HSMC)

Undertakes health service research, Kieran Walshe and Maria Dineen have a particular interest in research in clinical risk management, claims, clinical effectiveness and clinical governance.

Contact: Maria Dineen,
             Health Service Management Centre,
             Park House,
             40 Edgbaston Road,
             Birmingham,
             B15 2RT
             Tel: 0190 576 0788

Litigation & Risk Management Network

Objectives/Activities:
Comprises of Claims Managers, Risk Managers, Legal Service Managers, Health & Safety Managers and others with similar responsibilities for all types of Trusts and Health Authorities from Northern Yorkshire & Yorkshire and Trent Regions.

Meets quarterly at Pinderfields Hospital, Wakefield, to network, share problems and experiences, keep up to date with current topics, benchmark activities/procedures, hear guest speakers, etc.

Contact: Michael O'Connell,
Trust Administration Manager,
Pinderfields Hospitals NHS Trust,
Trust HQ,
Rowan House,
Pinderfields General Hospital,
Aberford Road,
Wakefield,
WF1 4EE
Tel: 0192 421 3842
Fax: 0192 481 4929

London Clinical Risk Forum
Objectives/Activities:
Informal gathering, open to any Risk Managers based in Central London who have a remit for clinical risk management. The principle objective is to share best practice and experiences openly.

Contact: Anita Dougall,
Clinical Risk Adviser,
Chelsea & Westminster Healthcare NHS Trust,
369 Fulham Road,
London SW10 9NH,
Tel: 0181 746 8000

Medical Defence Union
Clinical Risk Dept.,
192 Altrincham Road,
Sharston,
Manchester,
M22 4RZ
Tel: 0161 428 1234

Northern Risk Management Forum
Objectives/Activities:

➤ A forum for networking with colleagues involved in the field of risk management.

➤ Guest speakers on topics of interest to the forum.

➤ Sharing of experience in the field of risk management.

➤ Site visits and benchmarking opportunities.

Contact: Henry Stahr,
Centre for Advanced Inter-Professional Development,
Continuing Education Unit,
The University of Salford,
Salford,
M5 4WT.

Royal College of Anaesthetics
Catherine Arden, Director, Professional Standards Directorate contact for critical incident reporting.

STORM (Scottish Trust Officers in Risk Management)
Objectives/Activities:
Informal network of about 40 people, meeting occasionally to discuss matters of mutual interest.

Contact: Martin Jackson,
Head of Pharmacy/Risk Management,
Law Hospital NHS Trust,
Carluke,
Lanarkshire,
ML8 5ER
Tel: 01698 36100
Fax: 01698 376671

Welsh Risk Pool
Objectives/Activities:

▶ Administration of self-insurance pool for Wales, including clinical negligence and personal injury.

▶ Occasional courses/seminars on risk management.

Contact: Gren Kershaw,
Chief Executive,
Glam Clwyd DGH Trust,
Bodel Wyddan,
LL18 5UQ
Tel: 01745 584136

West Midlands Clinical Consortium

Contact: Maria Dineen,
          Health Services Management Centre,
          Park House,
          40 Edgbaston Road,
          Birmingham,
          B15 2RT
          Tel: 0190 576 0788

Yorkshire Clinical Risk Co-ordinators Group

Objectives/Activities:

▶ To share good practice.

▶ To provide a 'hands on', problem-solving approach for issues raised by members of the group.

▶ Information exchange between members.

▶ To ensure peer support for clinical risk co-ordinators.

▶ To facilitate standard setting for clinical risk issues within the membership of the group.

▶ To provide a focal point for all clinical risk issues.

▶ To identify training needs and stimulate or provide training and continued education.

Meet bi-monthly, with additional special interest groups as and when appropriate.

Contact: Julie Finch,
          Clinical Risk Co-ordinator,
          Bradford Hospitals NHS Trust,
          Bradford Royal Infirmary,
          Duckworth Lane,
          Bradford,
          BD9 6RJ
          Tel: 01274 364648

Journals/Books

Clinical Risk Management
Ed. Charles Vincent
Published by BMJ Publishing Group, 1995.

Medical Negligence & Clinical Risk: Trends And Developments 1998
Vivienne Harpwood
Published by Monitor Press Ltd.,
Suffolk House,
Church Field Road
Sudbury,
Suffolk CO10 6YA

Risk Management in the NHS
NHS Management Executive
Leeds: NHSME, 1993.

Clinical Risk
Publications Subscriptions Dept.
Royal Society of Medicine Press Ltd.,
1 Wimpole Street,
London,
W1M 8AE
Tel: 0171 290 2928

Health Care Risk Report
The Marketing Dept.,
The Eclipse Group,
18–20 Highbury Place,
London,
N5 1QP
Tel: 0171 354 5858
Fax: 0171 354 8106

Health Law for Healthcare Professionals
Concise and informative review of the latest legal, financial and administrative developments which dictate how organisations care for patients.
Monitor Press Ltd,
Suffolk House,
Church Field Road,
Sudbury,
Suffolk CO10 6YA
Tel: 01787 467223
Fax: 01787 881147

Medical Law Monitor

Monthly medico legal newsletter summarising the most pertinent and influential cases likely to affect strategic and operational decision making.
Monitor Press Ltd.,
Suffolk House,
Church Field Road,
Sudbury,
Suffolk CO10 6YA
Tel: 01787 467223
Fax: 01787 881147

Managing Medical Risk

Thames Media International Ltd.,
7 Courtrai Road,
London,
SE23 1PL
Tel: 0181 699 2220
Fax: 0181 699 3735

Courses

Clinical Risk Unit (CRU)

Since its inception in September 1995 the CRU training programme under Pippa Bark has run over 50 conferences and training sessions on clinical risk management. Individual training days have been on the following:

- An introduction to clinical risk management.
- Adverse incident reporting systems.
- Medical negligence law.
- Medical record keeping.
- Obstetrics.
- Risk management in complaints.
- Anaesthetics.
- Surgery.
- Mental Health.
- Orthopaedics.
- Accident and Emergency.
- Complaints handling in General Practice.

Some of these training days will be repeated in the 1998/99 year and we do local based talks introducing staff to some of the principles of risk management.

From January 1999 the CRU are joining with CHIME, the Centre for Health Informatics and Multiprofessional Education to run part-time postgraduate courses in clinical risk management. These will include:

> a certificate (one year)
>
> diploma (two years)
>
> masters degree (two years)

The course is aimed at medical, senior nurses and management with a minimum of 5 years experience in the health service and with some experience of risk management.

For further information contact: Pippa Bark,
Psychology Dept.,
Clinical Risk Unit,
1–19 Torrington Place,
University College London,
Gower Street,
London,
WC1E 6BT
Tel: 0171 504 5977
Fax: 0171 391 1647
email: p.bark@ucl.ac.uk

Capsticks Solicitors
Diploma in Risk Management
Contact: Capsticks Solicitors,
77/83 Upper Richmond Road,
London,
SW15 2TT
Tel: 0181 780 2211

Integrated Care Pathways:

ICPs 'amalgamate all the anticipated elements of care and treatment of all members of the multidisciplinary team, for a patient or client of a particular case-type or grouping within an agreed time frame, for the achievement of agreed outcomes. Any deviation from the plan is documented as a "variance"; the analysis of which provides information for the review of current practice'. (Johnson 1997, *Pathways of Care*, Blackwell Science)
or:

'An ICP determines locally agreed, multidisciplinary practice based on guidelines and evidence where available, for a specific patient/client group. It forms part or all of the clinical record, documents the care given and facilitates the evaluation of outcomes for continuous quality improvement.' (NPA 1998)

NB: many names for the pathway tool, including:

- Anticipated Recovery Pathways.
- Multidisciplinary Pathways of Care.
- Care Maps.
- Critical Care Pathways.
- Care Profiles.
- Collaborative Care Pathways.
- Pathways of Care.
- Care Pathways.

Organisations:

National Pathway Association (NPA)

Formed in the early 1990s with local networks of pathway users around the UK. In 1994 the networks met together to form the National Pathway User Group (NPUG), which at the time provided a simple network for members. October 1995, the NPUG became an official subscription based organisation with a committee to administer the membership and the national quarterly meetings. In 1997, the NPUG changed its name to the National Pathway Association (NPA), to include non-pathway users into the membership. Membership now in excess of 250 representing NHS Trusts from acute, community and mental health settings, primary care and private healthcare plus health authorities and purchasers.

Provides:

- quarterly newsletter
- membership/contact list
- quarterly national meetings.

Carole Cairns (membership secretary),
Priory Hospitals Group,
Broadwater Park,
Denham,
Uxbridge,
Middlesex UB9 5HP
Tel: 01895 836339
Website: available through the National Centre for Clinical Audit: www.ncca.org.uk and the address for the NPA pages within NCCA is: www.ncca.org.uk/nap1.htm

Scottish Pathway User Group

Network of pathway users across Scotland. Host national meetings three times a year, and publish newsletter. Membership is free. More recently the focus of this group has moved towards the evaluation and review of pathways already in place.
Provides:

 newsletter (3 times per year)

 national meetings (3 times per year)

 database of contacts for all members.

Clinical Audit Office,
West Glasgow Hospital,
Glasgow,
Scotland G11 6NT
Tel: 0141 211 2036

Journals, Periodicals, Books and Reports

The following gives an example of the many journals and texts that now include articles on Integrated Care Pathways and related topics.

Journals

Journal of Integrated Care

(formerly the Journal of Managed Care)
Editor: Harry Burns
The Royal Society of Medicine Press,
PO Box 9002,
London
W1A 0ZA
Tel: 0171 290 2927/8
Fax: 0171 290 2929
email: gayle.murray@roysocmed.ac.uk

Individual annual subscriptions £65 (Europe).
Institution annual subscriptions £120 (Europe).

NPA Newsletter

For members of the NPA.
Carole Cairns, etc., as above.

Reports

The Origins and Use of Care Pathways in the USA, Australia and the United Kingdom
Lynne Currie & Gill Harvey (1997),
Report No. 15,
Royal College of Nursing,
Dynamic Quality Improvement Programme,
RCN Institute,
Oxford Centre,
Radcliffe Infirmary,
Woodstock Road,
Oxford
OX2 6HE

International Journal of Health Care Quality Assurance
MCB University Press Ltd.,
60/62 Toller Lane,
Bradford,
West Yorkshire
BD8 9BY
Tel: 01274 777700
Fax: 01274 785200

Books

Pathways of Care
Edited Sue Johnson (1997),
Blackwell Science,
Osney Mead,
Oxford
OX2 OEL

Integrated Care Management; The Path to Success?
Edited Jo Wilson (1997),
Butterworth-Heinemann,
Linacre House,
Jordan Hill,
Oxford
OX2 8DP

Clinical Pathways Workbook

Sue Middleton and Adrian Roberts (1998),
Clinical Pathways Reference Centre,
VFM Unit,
Croesnewydd Hall,
Wrexham Technology Park,
Wrexham,
Wales LL13 7YP
Tel: 01978 727472
Fax: 01978 727470

Courses

No courses exist that give a professional qualification; most Integrated Care Pathway training exists as part of clinical audit, managed care or continuous quality improvement courses. However, some independent parties do provide regular training on ICPs.

▶ Basic Training in Care Pathways (1 day)

▶ Pathway Facilitator Training Course (3 days)

▶ Variance Tracking Training (1 day).

Sue Johnson Associates,
Primrose Cottage,
Old Odiham Road,
Alton,
Hampshire GU34 4BW
Tel: 0802 913289 (mobile)
Tel: 01420 543016

ICP Training,
VFM Unit,
Croesnewydd Hall,
Wrexham Technology Park,
Wrexham,
Wales LL13 7YP
Tel: 01978 727472
Fax: 01978 727470

National Pathway Association Quarterly National Meetings. All issues regarding ICP development and management considered. Carole Cairns, NPA, etc, as above.

▶ Care Pathway Seminars (1 day) every 6 months

Healthcare Risk Resources International Ltd.,
4th Floor,
40 Lime Street,
London
EC3M 5EA
Tel: 0171 220 7890
Fax: 0171 220 7891

Health Care Needs Assessment

Stevens and Raftery define healthcare need as 'the population's ability to benefit from healthcare'.[1] Information is commonly collected in three ways:

Epidemiological needs assessment published and local information on the incidence and prevalence of a disease, together with evidence of interventions effectiveness, are used to define the needs of the local population (i.e. how many people could benefit by how much from a given service). This is the gold standard for evidence-based practice. However, the information needed to complete an epidemiological needs assessment is not always available.

Comparative needs assessment compares services, activity and routine health data within and between districts to identify significant differences. When using this approach it is difficult to distinguish between what is needed, what is supplied and what is demanded.

Corporate needs assessment takes account of the opinions and wishes of local people, GPs, providers, national and regional policy makers and other agencies. Again, there may be a blurring of needs and demand.

Health Needs Assessment

Health needs assessment aims to assess the overall health of the community.[1] The community may be defined geographically, culturally or administratively such as a General Practice population. Commonly a three pronged approach is used.

▶ Collation of routine data on births, morbidity, use of health and social care services, mortality and social indicators, such as unemployment, which affect health.

▶ Establish the community's own assessment of their health and health needs, through questionnaires, individual interviews or focus groups.

▶ Ascertain the views of key individuals and organisations as to the health and health needs of the community.

Sources of information on needs assessment methodology

Books

Annett H and Rifkin SB. Guidelines for rapid participatory appraisal to assess community health needs: a focus for health improvements for low-income urban and rural areas. Geneva WHO. 1995.

Bie Nio Ong. Rapid appraisal and health policy. Ong Bie Nio 0412628201. London. Chapman & Hall. 1996. Buckingham Open University Press. 1966.

Dixon M, Murray T, Jenner D. (Eds) Radcliffe Medical Press (1977).

Fenner D and Pinchen I. Department of Health (1996).

Gillam SJ and Murray SA. Needs Assessment in General Practice. Occasional Paper 73. Royal College of General Practitioners. 1996.

Harris A. (Ed) Needs to know: A guide to needs assessment for primary care. Royal Society of Medicine Press (1997).

Hawtin M, Hughes G and Percy-Smith J. Open University Press (1994).

Last JM. A Dictionary of Epidemiology. 3rd Edition. Oxford University Press. 1995.

Mackintosh J, Bhopal R and Unwin N. Step by Step Guide to Epidemiological Health Needs Assessment for Ethnic Minority Groups. University of Newcastle.

Robinson J and Elkan R. Health needs assessment: theory and practice. Churchill Livingstone. 1996.

Sanderson HF, Mountney LM and Anthony PA. Casemix for All. Oxford Radcliffe Medical Press. 1998.

Stevens A and Raftery J. Healthcare needs assessment – the epidemiologically-based needs assessment reviews. Second Series. The Wessex Institute. Radcliffe Medical Press. 1997.

Wilkin D, Hallam L and Doggett M. Measures of needs and outcome for primary healthcare. Oxford Medical Publications. Oxford University Press. 1992.

Wright J. Health Needs Assessment in Practice. 1998.

Papers

Gillam S. Assessing the health needs of populations – the general practitioners contribution.
British Journal of General Practice. 1992; 42 at pp. 404–405.

Jordan J, Dowswell T, Harrison S and Lilford R. Whose Priority? Listening to users and the public. BMJ 1998; 316 at pp. 1668–1670.

Jordan J and Wright J. Making sense of health needs assessment. British Journal of General Practice. 1997; 48 at pp. 695–696.

Mackenzie I, Nelder R and Radford G. Needs assessment at a practice level; using routine data in a meaningful way. Journal of Public Health. Vol. 19 No. 3 at pp. 255–261.

Murray S and Graham L. Practice based health needs assessment: use of four methods in a small neighbourhood. BMJ 1995; 310 at pp. 1443–1448.

Royal College of Nursing. The GP practice population profiles: A framework for every member of the primary healthcare team. London RCN. 1993.

Ruta DA, Duffy MC and Farquharson A. Determining priorities for change in primary care: the value of practice based needs assessment. British Journal of General Practice. 1997; 47 at pp. 353–357.

Shanks J, Kheraj S and Fish S. Better ways of assessing health needs in primary care. BMJ. 1995; 308 at pp. 480–481.

Stevens A and Gabbay J. Needs Assessment Needs Assessment . . . Health Trends 1991; 23 (1) at pp. 20–21.

Stevens A and Gillam S. Needs Assessment from theory to practice. BMJ 1998. 316 at pp. 1448–1452.

Wilkinson M. Assessment in primary care: practical issues and possible approaches. BMJ 1998; 316 at pp. 1524–1528.

Williams R and Wright J. Epidemiological issues in health needs assessment. BMJ 1998; 316 at pp. 1379–1382.

Wright J, William R and Wilkinson J. Development and importance of health needs assessment. BMJ 1998; 316 at pp. 1310–1313.

NHS IMG Reference G7108. A Methodology for the Health Benefit Group Development Project. Available from The National Casemix Office, Information Management Group, NHS Executive Headquarters, Highcroft, Romsey Road, Winchester SO22 5DH. **Tel:** 01962 844 588.

NHS IMG Reference G7103. Health Benefit Group Development Project.

Wright J and Walley J. Assessing health needs in developing countries. BMJ 1998; 316 at pp. 1819–1823.

Organisations

Faculty of Public Health
4 St Andrews Place,
London NW1 4LB
Tel: 0171 224 0642

Public Health Forum
Contributions: John Fox, Office for National Statistics, 1 Drummond Gate, London SW1V 2QQ
Distribution: Katie Stone, King's Fund, 11–13 Cavendish Square, London W1M 0AN

Royal College of Nursing
20 Cavendish Square,
London W1M 9AE
Tel: 0171 409 3333

Association of Public Health
Trevelyan House,
30 Great Peter Street,
London SW1P 0HW
Tel: 0171 413 1896

The National Casemix Office,
Information Management Group,
NHS Executive Headquarters,
Highcroft, Romsey Road,
Winchester SO22 5DH
Tel: 01962 844 588

Faculty of Public Health Medicine.
http://www.his.path.cam.ac.uk/phealthy/fphm.htm

The First Report of the National Screening Committee.
This contains the criteria by which a screening test should be assessed.
http://www.open.gov.uk/doh/nsc/chap61.htm#criteria

Examples of Good Practice involving Patients.
http://www.open.gov.uk/doh/pcharter/phctip3.htm

Undertaking Systematic Reviews of Research on Effectiveness.
CRD Guidelines for Those Carrying Out or Commissioning Reviews.
CRD Report Number 4 January 1996.
http://www.york.ac.uk/inst/crd/report4.htm

Courses

Most universities run MSc courses in Public Health. Often these are modular allowing an individual to tailor the course of their own needs. The most well known course is at:

London School of Hygiene and Tropical Medicine,
Keppel Street,
London WC1E 7HT
Course organiser: Dr Aileen Clarke
Tel: 0171 636 8636

References

1   Stevens A and Raftery J. Healthcare needs assessment – the epidemiologically-based needs assessment reviews. The Wessex Institute. Radcliffe Medical Press Second series. 1997.
2   Gillam SJ and Murray SA. Needs Assessment in General Practice. Occasional Paper 73. Royal College of General Practitioners 1996.
3   Murray S and Graham L. Practice based health needs assessment: use of four methods in a small neighbourhood. BMJ 1995; 310 at pp. 1443–1448.

Index